Aids to Postgraduate Medicine

Aids to Postgraduate Medicine

J. L. Burton
MD BSc FRCP
Consultant Senior Lecturer in
Dermatology, Bristol Royal
Infirmary

FOURTH EDITION

CHURCHILL LIVINGSTONE
EDINBURGH LONDON MELBOURNE AND NEW YORK 1983

CHURCHILL LIVINGSTONE
Medical Division of Longman Group Limited

Distributed in the United States of America by
Churchill Livingstone Inc., 1560 Broadway, New
York, N.Y. 10036, and by associated companies,
branches and representatives throughout the
world.

First edition 1970
Second edition 1974
Third edition 1978
Fourth edition 1983

ISBN 0 443 02936 9

British Library Cataloguing in Publication Data
Burton, J. L.
    Aids to postgraduate medicine.—4th ed.
    1. Pathology   2. Medicine
    I. Title
    616   RB111

Library of Congress Cataloging in Publication Data
Burton, J. L. (John Lloyd)
    Aids to postgraduate medicine.
    Bibliography: p.
    Includes index.
    1. Internal medicine—Out lines, syllabi, etc.
    I. Title.
    RC59. B87   1983   616   82-17864

Printed in Singapore by Selector Printing Co Pte Ltd

Preface

This book is intended primarily to provide a compact aid to revision for candidates taking postgraduate examinations such as the M.R.C.P. (U.K.). I hope it will also prove useful to other doctors wishing quickly to refresh their memory of the diagnostic possibilities in a particular case.

This edition has been completely revised, and some new material has been added. Some of the lists have been derived from the textbooks named in the Bibliography, but the majority have come from the excellent review articles which now appear regularly in the journals and annual books devoted to postgraduate education. Many of the lists are followed by suggestions for further reading, so that this book should serve as a readily available source of reference to articles which will provide a comprehensive review as well as an introduction to the original literature.

I should like to thank the many people who have suggested improvements to this book, and I am particularly indebted to many of my colleagues in the Bristol Health District who have given me much helpful advice and constructive criticism.

1983   J.L.B.

Contents

The M.R.C.P. examination

The Royal College of Physicians held a Symposium in 1977 to explain some recent changes in the M.R.C.P. examination. The published proceedings (*Brit. Med. J.* 1978, 1: 217) may be summarized as follows:

The Part I examination. This is designed to filter off candidates who are insufficiently prepared for the Part II examination. Only about one-third of candidates pass the Part I examination each year.

Candidates are advised to prepare by wide reading of textbooks and monographs, particularly on the main themes relevant to clinical practice in Britain. Questions are asked about common and important topics, and also about areas of new knowledge.

Each paper has 60 questions, selected from a bank of about 4000 questions and over 100 new questions are added to the bank each year. The distribution of the 60 questions is as follows:

Cardiology	4	Clinical pharmacology	5
Respiratory	4	Symptoms and signs	1 or 2
Gastroenterology	4	Endocrinology	3
Tropical	1 or 0	Renal disease	3
Statistics	1	Muscular and skeletal	2
Anatomy	1	Reticuloendothelial	1
Physiology	1	Toxicology	1
Neurology	4	Immunology and allergy	1 or 2
Haematology	2 or 3	Industrial medicine	1
Dermatology	1	Metabolic disease	2
Venereology	1	Genetics	1
Paediatrics	4	Ophthalmology	1
Psychiatry	4	Infectious disease	2 or 3

The multiple true-false format is used, with five items in each question. The marking is +1 for a correct answer, −1 for a wrong answer, and 0 for 'don't know'. Candidates often look for subtlety that is not intended by the examiner and each question should be taken at its face value. Variation in standards from year to year is checked by using in each paper 6 to 10 marker questions which have been used before.

The Part II examination. Like Part I, this is a test of knowledge, but in addition it tests skill in history-taking and physical examination, judgement and attitudes (e.g. is the candidate kind and considerate?).

Essay questions are no longer used, because their marking is subjective and therefore unreliable. The present written paper can be objectively marked. Each question has an accepted answer, but the examiners are allowed to use their own judgement in giving appropriate marks if the candidate has given some other answer. Candidates have to answer questions on diagnosis and investigation following 4 case-histories (with no choice), and 10 data interpretations. The latter include electrocardiograms, but are mainly laboratory data. There are also questions on 20 projected slides (or pairs of slides). Each is shown for 90 seconds, after which a bell rings, and another 30 seconds is then allowed before the slide is changed. When slides of the fundi are shown, a picture of a normal fundus is first projected and photographic artefacts are pointed out.

The long case tests skill in history-taking and physical examination. The examiners recognize that the long case, especially the history, is probably the least valid part of the examination because so much depends on the individual patient. The short cases (usually only 3) probably give the examiners a better idea of the candidate's skill in physical examination. The candidate is examined by two examiners for 20 minutes on each occasion.

The oral examination is not simply a test of knowledge, but is supposed to find out how a candidate reacts to certain clinical situations and whether he understands basic principles. The oral examination has 2 examiners who each examine the candidate for 10 minutes. Specialist examiners (e.g. neurologists) do not take part in the oral examination.

Marks are allocated in the Part II examination in the proportion of two for the written paper, two for the clinical and one for the oral, but no candidate can pass if he fails the clinical examination.

Candidates can take the whole of Part II either in general medicine or in paediatrics.

A letter to *The Lancet* (July 25, 1981, p. 206) from the Presidents of the three Royal Colleges of Physicians (London, Glasgow and Edinburgh) made the following points. The primary purpose of the M.R.C.P. (U.K.) is to signify fitness to proceed to higher medical training as a physician. The candidate must therefore be competent in the basic skills of history-taking, physical examination, selection of tests and communication with patients. In recent years, increasing numbers of candidates, both from U.K. medical schools and overseas, have been found to be lacking these skills in some measure. For this reason the three Colleges now require, before candidates can be admitted to Part II of the examination, that they be qualified for 2½ years and that they have had a period of one year in acute medicine after preregistration appointments. The experience of acute medicine should be based on 'unselected' patients with a general range of clinical problems. Training programmes which involve rotation through a number of specialized units are acceptable, but the care of acutely-ill patients must represent a significant component of the appointments. The Colleges will depend heavily on the advice provided by the sponsors when application forms are being completed.

FURTHER READING

Cohen J A 1982 British Journal of Hospital Medicine 28: 361

Cardiology

AUSCULTATION

HEART SOUNDS

1. Valve closure
1st heart sound (mitral and tricuspid valves)
    (i) Loud in: Mitral stenosis
                Hyperdynamic circulation
                Tachycardia
   (ii) Normally split in tricuspid area on inspiration

2nd heart sound (aortic and pulmonary valves)
    (i) Normally split on inspiration, especially in children
   (ii) Loud narrowly split P_2 in pulmonary hypertension
 (iii) Soft widely split P_2 in pulmonary stenosis
 (iv) Widely split in RBBB
  (v) Widely split fixed P_2 in ASD
 (vi) Paradoxically split P_2 (narrows on inspiration) in LBBB and rarely in aortic stenosis and severe hypertension

2. Opening snap
Heard only with AV valve stenosis
Indicates mobile AV valve
Mitral opening snap in mitral stenosis is maximal medial to apex, louder during expiration, thereby differentiated from split P_2
Closeness to 2nd sound indicates severity of stenosis

3. Ejection sounds
Early systolic clicks due to aortic or pulmonary stenosis, or to dilatation of pulmonary artery or aorta in pulmonary or systemic hypertension. Mid-systolic clicks due to mitral valve prolapse.

4. Ventricular filling sounds (Triple rhythm)

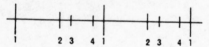

Diastolic sounds are due to:
    (i) 3rd heart sound (rapid ventricular filling)
    (ii) atrial (4th) sound (forceful atrial contraction)
    (iii) summation of both

3rd heart sound is normal in young people. Occurs in older people in:
    (i) R or L ventricular failure
    (ii) Mitral or tricuspid regurgitation
    (iii) Constrictive pericarditis (early and sharp)

Atrial sound is abnormal, occurs in resistance to LV filling e.g. hypertensive LVH, aortic stenosis
Summation sound is normal during tachycardia

5. Extracardiac sounds
Usually pericardial in origin, vary with respiration and posture

HEART MURMURS

High-pitched indicate large pressure difference across small orifice, e.g. AS
Low-pitched indicate small pressure difference across large orifice, e.g. MI

1. Systolic
    (i) Midsystolic ejection murmurs
        Aortic
        a. Aortic stenosis—confirmed by narrow pulse pressure and thrill (patient leaning forward in expiration)
        b. Increased flow rate
        c. Valve thickening or sclerosis without stenosis
        d. Post-valvar dilatation, e.g. hypertension or aortic aneurysm
        Pulmonary
        a. Functional, especially in young people
        b. Pulmonary stenosis
        c. Increased flow rate ASD, TAPVD (total anomalous pulmonary venous drainage), hyperdynamic circulation
        d. Post-valvar dilatation, e.g. pulmonary hypertension
    (ii) Pansystolic murmurs
        Extend from 1st to 2nd sound
        a. Mitral regurgitation—propagated into axilla
           (In mitral valve prolapse there may be a late systolic murmur).
        b. Tricuspid regurgitation—increases with inspiration, soft unless pulmonary hypertension is present
        c. VSD—3rd or 4th LICS. Thrill in 90%

Causes of a loud systolic murmur with a thrill
    (i) At apex—mitral regurgitation
   (ii) At 4th LICS—VSD
  (iii) At pulmonary area—pulmonary stenosis
  (iv) At aortic area—aortic stenosis

2. Diastolic

   (i) *Mitral or tricuspid stenosis*
      Degree of stenosis indicated by duration of murmur, not intensity
      Mitral stenosis—use bell, lightly applied at apex, with patient on L side in expiration. Presystolic accentuation is often a sign of pure stenosis, but is absent in atrial fibrillation
      Tricuspid stenosis—murmur louder on inspiration
   (ii) *Mitral or tricuspid thickening* e.g. Carey-Coombs murmur of active rheumatic carditis
  (iii) *Increased AV flow rate*
      Mitral in VSD and PDA (patent ductus arteriosus)
      Tricuspid in ASD and TAPVD
  (iv) *Aortic or pulmonary regurgitation*
      Aortic regurgitation—often missed. Listen with diaphragm all down L sternal edge for soft 'whispered R' murmur with patient learning forward in expiration
      Pulmonary regurgitation—usually due to pulmonary hypertension
      Austin-Flint murmur (functional mitral stenosis) may occur in Aortic Incompetence
      GrahaM-Steell murmur (pulmonary regurgitation) may occur in Mitral Stenosis with pulmonary hypertension

3. Continuous ('Machinery murmur')

    (i) Patent ductus arteriosus (2nd LICS or under clavicle)
   (ii) Aortico-pulmonary septal defect (2nd or 3rd LICS)
  (iii) Pulmonary AV fistula (over lung fields)
  (iv) Bronchial artery anastomosis in pulmonary atresia
   (v) Artificial ductus (Blalock or Waterston shunt)
  (vi) Venous hum

FURTHER READING

Hamer J 1979 Medicine, 3rd. series, 19: 951

Effect of respiration on murmurs
Inspiration increases stroke volume of R ventricle, therefore increases intensity of TS, TI and PS
Inspiration increases vascular volume of lungs and decreases stroke volume of L ventricle, therefore decreases intensity of MS, MI, AS and AI

Effect of posture on murmurs and cardiac sounds

Mitral systolic and diastolic murmurs. Accentuated in L lateral position

Aortic murmurs, ejection clicks and pericardial rub. Accentuated when sitting up

Functional systolic murmurs. Accentuated when lying down

Venous hum. Heard only when upright

Effect of drugs on murmurs
Drugs increasing arteriolar resistance will decrease systolic ejection murmurs and increase regurgitant murmurs at all valves
Vasodilators have the opposite effect

Characteristics of innocent systolic murmurs in childhood
1. No other abnormality detected
2. No thrill
3. Usually short, of low frequency, and in early or mid-systole
4. Not localised to a specific area, and not radiating outside praecordium
5. Intensity often varies with change in posture

FURTHER READING

Hamer J 1979 Medicine, 3rd series, 19: 951
Leatham A 1976 Auscultation of the heart and phonocardiography, 2nd edn. Churchill Livingstone, Edinburgh

CAUSES OF VALVULAR DISEASE

1. Congenital
2. Mitral valve prolapse (affects 5% of population)
3. Rheumatic
4. Syphilis
5. Infective endocarditis (bacterial or mycotic)
6. Libman-Sach's endocarditis (SLE)
7. Non-bacterial thrombotic endocarditis (usually with malignancy)

(contd)

8. Carcinoid
9. Ankylosing spondylitis
10. Marfan's
11. Atheroma
12. Dissecting aneurysm
13. Trauma

Differential diagnosis
1. Functional murmur
2. Atrial myxoma
3. Hypertrophic cardiomyopathy
4. Ruptured papillary muscle or chordae tendineae
5. Aneurysm of sinus of Valsalva

HEART FAILURE

VALSALVA MANOEUVRE

Normal response of pulse and BP

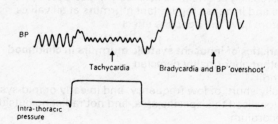

Cardiac failure causes a square wave response

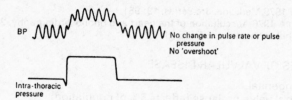

CAUSES OF LV FAILURE

1. **Pressure overload**
   (i) Hypertension
   (ii) Aortic stenosis
   (iii) Coarctation

2. **Volume overload**
   (i) Aortic or mitral regurgitation
   (ii) VSD or PDA
   (iii) AV fistula or anaemia

3. **Myocardial ischaemia**
   (i) Coronary artery disease
   (ii) Severe anaemia
   (iii) Tachycardia

4. **Primary myocardial disease**
   (i) Myocarditis
   (ii) Cardiomyopathy

CAUSES OF RV FAILURE

1. **Pressure overload**
   (i) Pulmonary hypertension secondary to LVF or MS
   (ii) Cor pulmonale
   (iii) Severe pulmonary stenosis

2. **Volume overload**
   (i) Tricuspid regurgitation
   (ii) ASD or TAPVD

FURTHER READING

Hamer J 1975 Medicine, 2nd series, 25: 1208

JUGULAR VENOUS PULSE

Normal jugular venous pulse wave

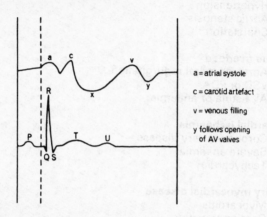

a = atrial systole

c = carotid artefact

v = venous filling

y follows opening of AV valves

Abnormalities of venous pulse wave
1. *Giant 'a' waves*
   (i) pulmonary hypertension
   (ii) severe pulmonary stenosis
   (iii) tricuspid stenosis
2. *Cannon waves*
   (i) Regular: Nodal rhythm
   (ii) Irregular: Complete heart block
        Multiple extrasystoles
3. *Absent 'a' waves:* atrial fibrillation
4. *Independent 'a' waves:* complete heart block
5. *Large 'v' waves:* tricuspid incompetence (confirm by palpation of systolic impulse in liver)
6. *Deep 'y' descent:* any cause of very high JVP especially constrictive pericarditis
7. *Slow 'y' descent:* tricuspid stenosis

CARDIAC CATHETERIZATION—Normal values

	Pressure (mmHg)
R. atrium	−1.5 to zero
R. ventricle	18/0 to 2
Pulmonary artery	18/8
Pulmonary 'wedge'	4
L. atrium	4
L. ventricle	130/0 to 10
Oxygen saturation of mixed venous blood (PA)	65–75%
Oxygen saturation of systemic arterial blood	96–98%

ARTERIAL PULSE

Causes of tachycardia
1. Sinus tachycardia (q.v.)
2. Supraventricular (atrial or nodal) tachycardia
3. Atrial flutter
4. Atrial fibrillation
5. Ventricular tachycardia
6. Ventricular flutter

Causes of sinus tachycardia
1. Hyperdynamic circulation (p. 20)
2. Congestive cardiac failure
3. Constrictive pericarditis
4. Drugs (adrenaline, atropine, nitrites, etc.)
5. Hypovolaemic shock (acute haemorrhage, etc.)

FURTHER READING

Besterman E 1975 Medicine, 2nd series, 25: 1200

Causes of a slow regular pulse
1. Sinus bradycardia (q.v.)
2. Complete heart block
3. 2 : 1 AV block
4. Atrial flutter or fibrillation with high degree of AV block
5. Sinus arrest with idionodal rhythm

Causes of sinus bradycardia
1. Congenital
2. Physical training
3. Convalescence from fever
4. Soon after myocardial infarction
5. Sinoatrial disorder ('sick sinus syndrome')
6. Jaundice
7. Myxoedema
8. Hypothermia
9. Raised intra-cranial pressure
10. Drugs (digitalis, betablockers, hypotensives)
11. Rapid rise in blood pressure
12. Transiently increased vagal tone (e.g. vomiting)

FURTHER READING

Shaw D 1979 Medicine, 3rd series, 19: 959

Causes of a 'dropped beat'
1. Sinoatrial block
2. Blocked atrial extrasystole
3. 2nd degree heart block

Causes of an irregular pulse
1. Extrasystoles (ventricular or supra-ventricular)
2. Atrial fibrillation
3. Sinus arrhythmia
4. Atrial flutter with varying block
5. 2nd degree heart block

Irregularity of volume also occurs in pulsus paradoxus and pulsus alternans

FURTHER READING

Bennett D H 1981 Cardiac arrhythmias-Practical notes on interpretation and treatment. J. Wright, Bristol

Causes of atrial fibrillation
1. Rheumatic heart disease, especially MS
2. Thyrotoxicosis
3. Myocardial ischaemia
4. Hypertension
5. Idiopathic ('lone') fibrillation, sick sinus syndrome or mitral valve prolapse
6. Chronic constrictive pericarditis
7. Atrial septal defect (over age 50)
8. Cardiomyopathy
9. Rarely atrial myxoma, bacterial endocarditis, acute pericarditis Ca bronchus, cor pulmonale, post-pneumonectomy, head injury

FURTHER READING

Evans T R 1979 British Journal of Hospital Medicine 21: 88

HEART BLOCK

Classification
1. Sinoatrial block
2. AV block
   1st degree, PR > 0.2 sec
   2nd degree
   (i) Dropped beats
       Fixed PR
       Varying PR (Wenkebach)
   (ii) Fixed AV relationship (2 : 1, 3 : 1, etc.)
   3rd degree, Complete
3. Bundle branch block
4. Intraventricular block

Causes
1. Congenital (usually AV nodal)
2. Idiopathic
3. Ischaemic heart disease
4. Aortic stenosis
5. Drugs (digitalis)
6. Cardiomyopathy (including myocardial infiltration and collagen-vascular disease)
7. Myocarditis (rheumatic, diphtheritic)
8. Rarely trauma, tumour, syphilis, hypertension

FURTHER READING

Shaw D 1979 Medicine, 3rd series, 19: 959

Wolff-Parkinson-White syndrome (short PR, widened QRS with recurrent paroxysmal tachycardia) is due to congenital accessory pathway for AV conduction with premature ventricular activation. Arrythmias caused by WPW syndrome
1. Paroxysmal tachycardia
2. Paroxysmal atrial fibrillation
3. Sinus node dysfunction

FURTHER READING

Camm J, Ward D 1979 Medicine, 3rd series, 19: 978

Sick sinus syndrome
There is considerable overlap between the physiological bradycardia seen in athletes, and that occurring in patients with the sick sinus syndrome, and profound bradycardia and even sinus arrest can occur in normal young people.

Definition of established sinoatrial disorder
A chronic sinus rate below 50 with one or more of the following:
1. Sinus pause of 2 seconds or more
2. Atrial rate below 40 (usually with junctional rhythm).
3. Paroxysmal tachycardia (AF., atrial flutter or atrial or ventricular tachycardia).

Potential sinoatrial disorder
A chronic unexplained sinus bradycardia in the absence of the above factors.

FURTHER READING

Shaw D B, Evans R C 1981 Journal of Royal College of Physicians 15: 179

ARTERIAL HYPERTENSION

Causes of pulmonary hypertension
1. *Passive*
   Secondary to raised L atrial pressure (MS or LVF)
2. *Hyperdynamic*
   L to R shunt (ASD, VSD, PDA and TAPVD)
3. *Reactive*
   (i) Vasoconstriction secondary to hypoxia
       High altitude
       Chronic bronchitis
       Kyphoscoliosis
       Upper respiratory tract obstruction
       Respiratory depression
   (ii) Obstructive
       Pulmonary thrombi or emboli
       Arteritis
       Parasites, e.g. schistosomiasis

Causes of systemic hypertension
A *Essential*
B *Secondary*
1. Renal
   (i) Ischaemia (esp. renal artery stenosis)
   (ii) Diffuse renal disease

2. Hormonal
    (i) Phaeochromocytoma
    (ii) Cushing's
    (iii) Oral contraceptives (increase angiotensin precursor)
    (iv) Primary aldosteronism (Conn's)
    (v) Acromegaly
3. Coarctation
4. Polycythaemia vera
5. Toxaemia of pregnancy
6. Neurogenic, e.g. head injury
7. Acute intermittent porphyria
8. ? Aortic valve homograft
9. ? Alcoholism

FURTHER READING

Pentecost B 1979 Medicine, 3rd series, 21: 1081

Drugs which may induce hypertension
1. Oestrogens and oral contraceptives
2. Corticosteroids
3. Sympathomimetics (e.g. phenylpropranolamine in 'cold cures')
4. Carbenoxolone, liquorice
5. Clonidine overdose or withdrawal
6. Drug interactions, e.g. guanethidine with tricylic
   antidepressants or indomethacin or methylamphetamine

FURTHER READING

Pearson R M, Havard C W H 1978 British Journal of Hospital Medicine
    20: 447

CARDIOMYOPATHY

The definition varies but some authorities restrict the term to heart
disease of unknown cause. Most authors exclude ischaemia (e.g.
anaemia) and valvular disease (e.g. carcinoid). Note that
hypertension is the only feature which distinguishes 'hypertensive
heart disease with failure' from 'congestive cardiomyopathy'.

CAUSES OF CARDIOMYOPATHY

A. Primary
1. *Hypertrophic (with or without a gradient)*
   Recent work suggests this condition is not obstructive
2. *Congestive (dilated)*
   Isolated cardiomegaly, gallop rhythm and idiopathic heart failure

   These two types account for 98% of primary cases in U.K.
3. *Restrictive*
   Endomyocardial fibrosis. May progress to the obliterative form.

B. Secondary
1. *Infective*
   (i) Viral (post-myocarditis)
   (ii) Bacterial, e.g. diphtheria toxin
   (iii) Protozoal, e.g. schistosomiasis
                       toxoplasmosis
                       trypanosomiasis (Chagas')
2. *Metabolic and endocrine*
   (i) Pregnancy and puerperium
   (ii) Hyperthyroidism, hypothyroidism, hypoadrenalism, acromegaly
   (iii) Haemochromatosis, glycogen storage disease (Pompe's), gargoylism (Hurler's), porphyria
   (iv) Thiamine deficiency (beri-beri)
   (v) Amyloidosis
3. *Neuromuscular*
   (i) Muscular dystrophy, especially Duchenne's and dystrophia myotonica
   (ii) Friedreich's ataxia
4. *Vasculitis* (including Löffler's disease)
5. *Leukaemia or granulomatous infiltrate (sarcoidosis)*
6. *Allergic*, e.g. serum sickness
7. *Drugs and chemicals*
   (i) Metals—cobalt, antimony, arsenic
   (ii) Alcohol
   (iii) Emetine
   (iv) Phenothiazine and tricyclic antidepressants
   (v) Anaesthetics
8. *Radiation*

C. Unclassified or indeterminate cardiomyopathy
1. Arrhythmia
2. Disorder of conducting tissue (e.g. familial heart block)
3. Prolapsing mitral valve
4. Angina with normal coronary vessels

FURTHER READING

Evan T 1979 Medicine, 3rd series, 20: 1042

COMPLICATIONS OF MYOCARDIAL INFARCTION
1. Cardiac arrhythmia: Almost any, but particularly—
    (i) Sinus bradycardia often with nodal escape
    (ii) Supraventricular tachycardia, atrial flutter, atrial fibrillation
    (iii) Ventricular tachycardia, flutter or fibrillation
    (iv) Heart block (all degrees)
    (v) Cardiac asystole
2. LVF
3. Hypotension and 'shock'
4. Pulmonary embolism (usually from leg veins)
5. Mural thrombus and systemic emboli
6. Pericarditis
7. Ruptured papillary muscle (causing mitral regurgitation)
8. VSD
9. Cardiac aneurysm or rupture
10. Dressler's syndrome (with late onset pleuro-pericarditis)
11. Psychological, including 'L. chest pain'
12. Frozen shoulder and 'shoulder hand' syndrome
13. Iatrogenic; drugs, pacing, etc.

FURTHER READING

Hampton J R 1977 British Journal of Hospital Medicine 17: 242
Mogensen L 1979 Medicine, 3rd series, 20: 1058

Causes of generalised cardiomegaly on chest X-ray
1. Congestive cardiac failure
2. Multiple valve lesions
3. Pericardial effusion
4. Cardiomyopathy
5. Myocarditis
6. Ebstein's disease
7. Hyperdynamic circulation
8. Complete heart block

CAUSES OF SYNCOPE
(Transient loss of consciousness, usually due to inadequate cerebral blood flow or hypoxaemia)

1. **Vasovagal**
   (i) Emotion, heat, standing still
   (ii) Loss of blood or plasma, dehydration
   (iii) Carotid sinus hypersensitivity
   (iv) Postural hypotension
        Prolonged recumbency
        Vasodilator drugs
        Autonomic neuropathy: familial, diabetes, etc.
        Micturition syncope

2. **Cardiac**
   (i) Cardiac standstill-vagal inhibition
   (ii) Stokes-Adams (heart block)
   (iii) Ventricular tachycardia or fibrillation
   (iv) Aortic stenosis, hypertrophic cardiomyopathy
   (v) Cyanotic cong. heart disease (fall in pO_2)
   (vi) Cough syncope (obstructed venous return)
   (vii) Massive pulmonary embolism
   (viii) Massive haemopericardium
   (ix) Atrial myxoma, ball-valve thrombus
   (x) Cardiogenic 'shock' (myocardial infarct)

3. **Vascular defect**
   (i) Carotid or vertebro-basilar insufficiency
        Atheroma, thrombosis, embolism
        Migraine
        Cervical spondylosis, strangulation, etc.
   (ii) Subclavian steal syndrome

4. **Hypoxaemia**
e.g., high altitude, anaemia
For other causes of coma, see page 109

FURTHER READING

Fowler T 1982 British Journal of Hospital Medicine 27: 224

CARDIAC ARREST

Causes
1. Myocardial ischaemia
2. Hypoxia (e.g. in anaesthesia)
3. Vagal reflexes (e.g. carotid sinus)
4. Hyperkalaemia
5. Hypothermia
6. Hypercapnia
7. Electrocution
8. Drugs, e.g. digitalis, quinidine, adrenaline
9. Diagnostic procedures (cardiac catheterization, bronchoscopy, etc.)
10. Severe hypotension
11. Massive pulmonary embolism

FURTHER READING

Rowlands D J 1976 British Journal of Hospital Medicine 15: 312

'SHOCK'

Clinical shock may be defined as a syndrome where inadequate blood supply and elimination of tissue metabolites lead to functional and/or structural disturbances in essential organs.

Causes of clinical shock
1. *Hypovolaemia*
   Haemorrhage, trauma, dehydration, burns
2. *Cardiac failure*
   (i) Pump failure
   (ii) Arrhythmia
   (iii) Obstruction (e.g. pulmonary embolism)
3. *Sepsis*
4. *Anaphylaxis*

FURTHER READING

Joseph S P 1976 British Journal of Hospital Medicine 16: 349
Resnekov L 1977 British Journal of Hospital Medicine 17: 232

CAUSES OF PERICARDITIS

1. Infective
   (i) Viral
   (ii) Bacterial (pyogenic or TB)
   (iii) Fungal
   (iv) Parasitic
2. Rheumatic fever
3. Collagen-vascular, especially SLE
4. Cardiovascular
   (i) Myocardial infarction
   (ii) Post infarction syndrome
   (iii) Post-cardiotomy syndrome
   (iv) Aortic dissection
   (v) Endomyocardial fibrosis
5. Neoplasm, especially bronchial carcinoma
6. Metabolic
   (i) Uraemia
   (ii) Hypothyroidism
   (iii) Hyperuricaemia
7. Trauma
8. Drugs (phenylbutazone, procainamide, practalol)
9. Radiation
10. Idiopathic (probably viral)

FURTHER READING

Brigden W 1979 British Journal of Hospital Medicine 21: 7
Cobbe S M 1980 British Journal of Hospital Medicine 23: 250
Flavell G 1979 Bristish Journal of Hospital Medicine 21: 21
Hollman A 1975 Medicine, 2nd series, 29: 1393

CAUSES OF HYPERDYNAMIC CIRCULATION

1. Exercise or emotion (anxiety, fright, etc.)
2. Pregnancy
3. Anaemia
4. Pyrexia
5. Thyrotoxicosis
6. AV aneurysm
7. Paget's disease
8. Beri-beri
9. Hepatic failure
10. Hypercapnia
11. Erythroderma
12. Vasodilator drugs

ELECTROCARDIOGRAPHY

Cardiac axis

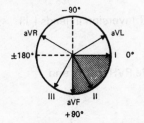

Leads with the maximum
positive deflection
indicate the cardiac axis

Normal axis is 0° to + 90°
Right axis deviation is + 90° to + 180°
Left axis deviation is 0° to – 120°
(But axis of 0° to – 30° may occur in stocky build, pregnancy and
ascites)

Ventricular hypertrophy

Minimal criteria for LVH
Either R in aVL > 13 mm
Or R in V5 or 6 > 27 mm
Or S in V1 + R in V5 or 6 > 35 mm, providing the circulation is not
hyperdynamic

Minimal criteria for RVH
Rs or qR complex in V1 or V3r with ventricular activation time >
0.03 sec, QRS < 0.12 sec, and R axis deviation

Combined LVH and RVH
Signs of LVH in precordial leads with a frontal plane axis of more
than + 90°

FURTHER READING

Hamer J 1978 An introduction to electrocardiography, 2nd edn. Pitman,
Tunbridge Wells

ECG signs of infarction
1. *Antero-septal*
Pathological Q and/or ST elevation and T inversion in leads I, a VL
and V1–4

2. *Antero-lateral*
Pathological Q and/or ST elevation and T inversion in leads I, aVL and V4–6

3. *Inferior* (*diaphragmatic*)
Pathological Q and/or ST elevation and T inversion in leads I, III and aVF

4. *True Posterior*
Tall R waves in leads V1 and V2. (Exclude RVH, RBBB and Wolff-Parkinson-White)

5. *Subendocardial*
ST depression and T inversion in overlying leads, with reciprocal ST elevation and upright T in leads from the opposite surface and in cavity leads

FURTHER READING

Rowley J M, Hampton J R 1981 British Journal of Hospital Medicine 26: 253

Causes of low T waves
 1. Thick chest wall or emphysema
 2. Pericardial effusion
 3. Ischaemia
 4. Myocarditis or cardiomyopathy
 5. Constrictive pericarditis
 6. Hypothyroidism, hypopituitarism or hypoadrenalism
 7. Non-penetrating chest trauma
 8. Drugs—digitalis, quinidine
 9. Hypokalaemia or hypocalcaemia
10. Abdominal visceral disease, e.g. pancreatitis, cholecystitis
11. Post-tachycardia
12. Physiological
     (i) Juvenile pattern (esp. in Negroes)
    (ii) Eating a large meal or swallowing ice
   (iii) Anxiety
    (iv) Delirium tremens
     (v) Hyperventilation

FURTHER READING

Goldberg M J 1975 In: Lant A F (ed) Advanced medicine, symposium 11. Pitman, London, p 322

Causes of LBBB
1. Ischaemic heart disease
2. Hypertension
3. Aortic valve disease
4. Cardiomyopathy
5. Myocarditis

Causes of RBBB
1. Normal (especially in young people)
2. RV strain (especially pulmonary embolism)
3. ASD (especially ostium secundum)
4. Myocardial ischaemia
5. Myocarditis

ECG changes of hyperkalaemia
Tall T
Prolonged PR
Flattened P
Wide QRS
May be ventricular tachycardia or fibrillation

ECG changes of hypokalaemia
Flattened T
Prolonged PR
Depressed ST
Tall U
Hypercalcaemia:shortens QT
HyPOcalcaemia: PrOlongs QT

Chest disease

LUNG ANATOMY

BRONCHO-PULMONARY SEGMENTS

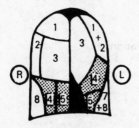

Anterior

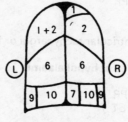

Posterior

Right lung
Upper lobe
1. Apical
2. Posterior
3. Anterior

Middle lobe
4. Lateral
5. Medial

Lower lobe
6. Apical
7. Medial basal
8. Anterior basal
9. Lateral basal
10. Posterior basal

Left lung
Upper lobe
1 & 2. Apico-posterior
3. Anterior
4. Superior lingular
5. Inferior lingular

Lower lobe
6. Apical
7 & 8. Antero-medial basal
9. Lateral basal
10. Posterior basal

LUNG MARKINGS

Upper border of lower lobe (oblique fissure). 2nd thoracic spine posteriorly to 6th rib in mammary line

Upper border of (R) middle lobe (transverse fissure). Horizontal line from 4th rib at sternum to the above line

Inferior border of lungs. 8th rib in mid-axillary line

PHYSIOLOGY

SPIROMETRY

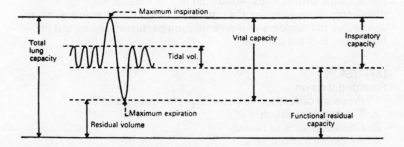

The resting expiratory level is the most constant reference point on the spirometer tracing

Minute ventilation
Product of tidal volume and number of respirations per minute

Vital capacity
Largest volume a subject can expire after a single maximal inspiration. Normal values increase with size of subject and decrease with age (about 4½ litres in young adult male). Can be reduced in practically any lung or chest wall disease

Forced vital capacity (FVC)
The vital capacity when the expiration is performed as rapidly as possible

FEV_1 (Forced expiratory volume in one second)
Volume expired during first second of FVC

Ratio $\dfrac{FEV_1}{FVC}$ should be 75% or more, and is reduced in obstructive airway diseases (asthma, emphysema, bronchitis)

Peak flow
Maximum expiratory flow rate achieved during a forced expiration. A convenient way to detect a reduction in ventilatory function. Also useful for serial measurements in the same patient and for assessing response to bronchial antispasmodics

Residual volume
Obtained by subtracting expiratory reserve volume from functional residual capacity. Residual volume is normally 20 to 25% of total lung capacity but increases in elderly, and in over-inflation of the lungs (emphysema, asthma)

Anatomical dead space
The volume of air in the mouth, pharynx, trachea and bronchi up to the terminal bronchioles (about 150 ml). In disease the physiological dead space may greatly exceed the anatomical dead space due to disorders of the ventilation/perfusion ration, but in health the two are identical

DIFFUSION
Rate depends on:
1. Pressure difference between alveolar gas and RBC
2. Thickness of tissue
3. Characteristics of tissue
4. Available surface area

Diffusion defects
Carbon dioxide is about 20 times more diffusible than oxygen. In diffusion defects the *arterial pO_2* is normal or slightly reduced at rest, but decreases markedly after exercise due to increased tissue uptake of O_2. *Arterial pCO_2* is normal or even reduced at rest (due to hyperventilation) and tends to fall on exercise

Diffusing capacity
Expressed as ml/min/mmHg pressure difference (or mmol/min/kPa)
May be reduced in:
1. Alveolo-capillary block
    (i) pulmonary oedema
    (ii) pulmonary fibrosis
    (iii) infiltrative lesions, e.g. sarcoidosis and lymphangitis carcinomatosa
2. Reduction in area available for diffusion
    (i) emphysema
    (ii) multiple pulmonary emboli
    (iii) pneumonectomy, cysts, etc.

3. Anaemia
May be increased in:
1. Increased pulmonary capillary bed
2. Polycythaemia

Compliance
The volume change produced by unit change of pressure, expressed as litres/cm. H_2O (or l/kPa)

Pulmonary compliance
A measure of lung elasticity. It is reduced when the lungs are abnormally stiff due to pulmonary venous congestion or infiltrative or fibrotic lesions of the lungs. It is increased in emphysema

Thoracic cage compliance
Decreased in kypho-scoliosis, skeletal muscle spasticity and pectus excavatum

FURTHER READING

Clarke S 1976 British Journal of Hospital Medicine 15: 137
Freedman S 1981 Hospital Update 7: 281
Saunders K B 1975 British Journal of Hospital Medicine, 14: 228

Causes of hypoventilation
1. Respiratory centre depression
   (i) Drugs
   (ii) Anoxia
   (iii) Hypercapnia
   (iv) Trauma
   (v) Raised IC pressure
   (vi) Primary alveolar hypoventilation
        (Pickwickian syndrome, with obesity and hypoventilation)
2. Neural or neuromuscular cause
3. Respiratory muscle disease
4. Limited thoracic movement
   (i) Kyphoscoliosis
   (ii) Elevated diaphragm
5. Limited lung movement
   (i) Pleural effusion
   (ii) Pneumothorax
6. Lung disease
   (i) Obstruction in upper or lower respiratory tract
   (ii) Atelectasis, pneumonia, etc.

Causes of hyperventilation
1. Anxiety, hysteria, pain
2. CNS lesions: meningitis, encephalitis, trauma, CVA, etc.
3. Drugs: salicylates, analeptics, adrenaline
4. Increased metabolism: hyperthyroidism, fever, etc.
5. Anoxia
6. Metabolic acidosis
7. Pulmonary reflexes: Irritant gases, pneumothorax, atelectasis, left ventricular failure
8. Hypotension
9. Artificial ventilation

FURTHER READING

West J B 1977 Ventilation. Blood flow and gas exchange, 3rd edn. Blackwell Scientific, Oxford

PHYSICAL SIGNS

CRACKLES AND WHEEZES

Crackles
Crackles (formerly called râles, moist sounds or crepitations) are non-musical lung sounds of short duration. Inspiratory crackles are produced by abrupt opening of closed airways in regions of the lung deflated to residual volume. Early inspiratory crackles are associated with severe airways obstruction, late inspiratory crackles with a restrictive defect due to fibrosis, infiltration or oedema.

Friction between the two layers of the pleura can also produce crackles, but they are usually louder, localized and occur in expiration as well as inspiration.

Wheezes
Wheezes (formerly called rhonchi) are musical lung sounds produced by air passing at high velocity through an airway narrowed to the point of closure. The pitch of the wheeze is determined by the velocity of the air-jet and is independent of the calibre and length of the airway. Thus in severe airway obstruction wheeze may be absent if ventilation is so reduced that the air-jet slows below the critical minimum velocity.

FURTHER READING

Forgacs P 1967 Lancet 2: 203
Nath A R, Capel L H 1974 Thorax 29: 223

COMMONLY CONFUSED SIGNS

Percussion
Skodaic resonance: hyperresonance above a pleural effusion level

Amphoric resonance: selective reinforcement of low-pitched vibrations by a cavity or pneumothorax

Cracked-pot sound: due to large cavity in communication with a bronchus

Vocal resonance
Whispering pectoriloquy: greatly increased vocal resonance, e.g. above a pleural effusion level

Aegophony: bleating sound heard occasionally above a pleural effusion level

Hippocratic succussion
Splashing noise due to gas and fluid in a cavity

Post-tussive suction
Sucking noise due to cavity springing open after a cough

EMPHYSEMA

Is characterised by enlargement of the air-spaces distal to the terminal bronchioles, either from dilatation or destruction of their walls. Some authorities (e.g. WHO and American Thoracic Society) restrict the term to conditions accompanied by tissue destruction.

THE EMPHYSEMA—CHRONIC BRONCHITIS SPECTRUM

	Emphysema ('Pink Puffers')	Chronic Bronchitis ('Blue Bloaters')
Course	Relentlessly progressive dyspnoea	Intermittent dyspnoea with exacerbations
Sputum	Scanty	Profuse, mucopurulent
Cor pulmonale	Infrequent, usually terminal	Frequent and remittent
Polycythaemia	Uncommon	Common
CXR	Attenuated peripheral vessels	Normal peripheral vessels
Arterial pCO$_2$	Normal	Raised
Alveolar gas transfer	Reduced	Normal

CAUSES OF EMPHYSEMA

Localised
1. Congenital
2. Compensatory, due to lung collapse, scarring or resection
3. Partial bronchial occlusion
   (i) foreign body
   (ii) neoplasm
   (iii) peribronchial lymphadenopathy (e.g. TB)
4. Rarely unilateral emphysema due to bronchiolitis before age 8 years (Macleod's syndrome).

Generalised
1. Idiopathic ('Primary')
2. Associated with chronic bronchitis, chronic asthma or pneumoconiosis } usually centrilobular
3. Senile (physiological)
4. Familial (some due to α_1 anti-trypsin deficiency, when the disease is usually basal)

FURTHER READING

Flenley D C 1978 Lancet 1: 542
Hugh-Jones P 1973 In: Walker G (ed) Advanced medicine, Symposium 9. Pitman, London, p 300
Reid L 1975 Hospital Update 1: 115

HARMFUL EFFECTS OF CIGARETTE SMOKING

1. *Pharmacological effects of nicotine*
   (i) CVS: rise in BP, tachycardia, cutaneous vasoconstriction
   (ii) Autonomic: transient stimulation, followed by depression of all ganglia
   (iii) Adrenal: discharges adrenaline
   (iv) CNS: stimulation, especially respiratory, vasomotor and emetic centres
   (v) Antidiuretic: due to ADH release

2. *Pharyngeal and bronchial irritation*
   (i) Bronchitis
   (ii) Post-op. pneumonia, etc.

3. *Carcinoma incidence increased*
   (i) Bronchus
   (ii) Oesophagus
   (iii) Prostate
   (iv) Bladder

4. *Cardio-vascular disease exacerbated*
   (i) Myocardial ischaemia
   (ii) Buerger's

5. *Peptic ulcer mortality increased*
   (but *not* incidence)

6. *Idiosyncrasy*
   (i) Tobacco angina
   (ii) Atrial extrasystoles
   (iii) Hypoglycaemia, etc.

7. *Tobacco amblyopia*
   (very rarely)

8. *Cirrhosis incidence increased*
   (probably due to associated alcoholism)

9. *Effect on fetus*
   Smoking during pregnancy restricts fetal growth and increases
   perinatal mortality rate

FURTHER READING

Third Report of Royal College of Physicians of London 1977 'Smoking or
   Health?' Pitman, London

CAUSES OF CHRONIC COR PULMONALE

1. Chronic bronchitis or emphysema.
2. Chronic asthma.
3. Bronchiectasis.
4. Pulmonary fibrosis (p. 33)
5. Pulmonary thromboembolism.
6. Kyphoscoliosis.
7. Chronic neuromuscular disease affecting chest.
8. Primary alveolar hypoventilation (including Pickwickian
   syndrome).

FURTHER READING

White R 1975 Medicine, 2nd series 26: 1336

INDUSTRIAL CHEST DISEASE

1. *Mineral dust pneumoconiosis*
Coal dust, silicates (including talc, kaolin and asbestos), iron, tin, tungsten, aluminium, etc.

2. *Disease due to organic dust*
Byssinosis, farmer's lung, bagassosis, mushroom-worker's lung, paprika-splitter's lung, etc.

3. *Disease due to industrial gases and fumes*
Manganese pneumonitis, cadmium emphysema, silo-filler's disease, metal fume fever (ZnO), etc.

4. *Occupational lung cancer*
Nickel-refining, chromate workers, retort-house workers in gasworks, asbestos workers, etc.

5. *Chronic bronchitis*
Many heavy, dusty industries

FURTHER READING

Horne N W 1976 British Journal of Hospital Medicine 15: 440
Seaton A 1979 Medicine, 3rd series, 24: 1224

CAUSES OF SLOW RESOLUTION OF PNEUMONIA

1. *Bronchial obstruction*
Neoplasm, foreign body (especially pea-nut), etc.

2. *Inappropriate chemotherapy*
Especially for staphylococcus, klebsiella, TB, mycosis

3. *Decreased host resistance*
Cachexia, agranulocytosis, immunoglobulin defects, LVF, etc.

4. *Pharyngeal pouch with 'spilling'*

5. *Formation of abscess, empyema or serous effusion*

6. *Other causes of pulmonary fibrosis* (p. 33)

CAUSES OF PULMONARY FIBROSIS

1. *Infections*
Especially TB, mycosis, varicella, psittacosis

2. *Pneumoconiosis*
Inorganic
  Silica, asbestos, talc, kaolin, tungsten, iron, Be, Al, china-clay
  Coal dust, but only in progressive massive fibrosis or Caplan's
  syndrome.

3. *Extrinsic allergic alveolitis*
Farmers, bird-fanciers, cheese-washers, malt-workers, etc., and
bagassosis

4. *Fibrosing Alveolitis*
Including rheumatoid lung and desquamative interstitial
pneumonitis

5. *Sarcoidosis*

6. *Aspiration*
Especially lipoid pneumonitis

7. *Cardiac*
Pulmonary oedema, mitral stenosis ossification, multiple
pulmonary infarcts, 'uraemic lung'

8. *Drugs and poisons*
Cytotoxic, e.g. busulphan.
Others, e.g. nitrofurantoin, paraquat

9. *Neoplastic*
Alveolar cell carcinoma, lymphangitis carcinomatosa

10. *Miscellaneous*
Systemic sclerosis, SLE, radiation, eosinophilic granuloma,
tuberous sclerosis (epiloia), xanthomatosis, biliary cirrhosis,
hypogammaglobulinaemia

When shown a chest radiograph with widespread miliary densities,
do not offer pneumoconiosis as a first suggestion if breast shadows
are visible

FURTHER READING

Turner-Warwick M 1974 British Medical Journal 2: 371
Scadding J G 1974 Thorax 29: 271
Stableforth D E 1979 British Journal of Hospital Medicine 22: 128

LUNG DISEASE CAUSED BY ASPERGILLUS

1. Asthma
2. Extrinsic allergic alveolitis (e.g. in maltworkers)
3. Aspergilloma
4. Invasive aspergillosis
5. Bronchopulmonary eosinophilia (q.v.)

FURTHER READING

Davies R J 1979 British Journal of Hospital Medicine 21: 136

Bronchopulmonary eosinophilia
1. *Eosinophilic bronchitis*
    (i) Uncomplicated asthma
    (ii) Asthma with casts, partial collapse and Aspergillus hypersensitivity
    (iii) As (ii), but with no Aspergillus hypersensitivity
2. *Eosinophilic pneumonia*
    (i) Parasitic, e.g. Ascaris (localized) or microfilariae (diffuse)
    (ii) Fungal, e.g. Aspergillus infection
    (iii) Drugs, e.g. nitrofurantoin, PAS., phenylbutazone
    (iv) Occupational, e.g. epoxy resins
    (v) Idiopathic ('prolonged pulmonary eosinophilia').
N.B. Polyarteristis nodosa is now regarded as a separate entity.

FURTHER READING

Grant I W B 1982 Hospital Update 8: 491

DRUG-INDUCED PULMONARY DISEASES

Drug	Pulmonary effect
1. Beta-blockers, aspirin, disodium cromoglycate	Asthma (pharmacological)
2. Many drugs, e.g. penicillin	Asthma (type I allergy)
3. Cytotoxics (esp. busulphan), ganglion-blockers	Fibrosing alveolitis
4. Pituitary snuff	Allergic alveolitis
5. Methotrexate	Granulomatous pneumonitis
6. Nitrofurantoin	Pulmonary eosinophilia with pleural effusion
7. Methysergide	Fibrosis and chronic pleural effusion
8. Procainamide, phenytoin, hydrallazine, isoniazid, etc.	Lupus erythematosus
9. Sulphonamides, etc.	Vasculitis
10. Heroin, methadone	Pulmonary oedema
11. Aminorex	Pulmonary hypertension
12. High conc. oxygen	Pneumonitis
13. Mineral oil (aspiration)	Pneumonitis or granuloma

Other drugs have indirect adverse effects on the lungs
1. *Infection* (esp. opportunistic or TB) due to glucocorticoids or cytotoxic drugs

2. *Aspiration* e.g. due to oversedation

3. *Pulmonary embolism* e.g. due to thrombophlebitis

4. *Bleeding* e.g. due to anticoagulants

FURTHER READING

Pritchard J 1979 Medicine, 3rd series, 23: 1254
Rosenow E C 1972 Annals of Internal Medicine 77: 977

CAUSES OF LUNG ABSCESS
1. Malignancy
(i) Necrotic bronchial carcinoma
(ii) Secondary to bronchial obstruction
(iii) Spill-over of pus or slough

2. Aspiration
  (i) Oral or pharyngeal sepsis
  (ii) Pharyngeal pouch
  (iii) Oesophageal obstruction, tracheo-oesophageal fistula
  (iv) Drowning
  (v) Bronchiectasis elsewhere in lung
  (vi) Coma, anaesthesia, alcoholic debauch, etc.

3. Vascular embolus
  (i) Secondary infection of pulmonary infarct
  (ii) Septic embolic due to pyaemia

4. Specific abscesses
  (i) Staphylococcal
  (ii) Friedlander's (klebsiella)
  (iii) TB
  (iv) Actinomycosis and other fungi
  (v) Entamoeba histolytica

5. Bronchial obstruction
Benign tumour, foreign body, mucoviscidosis, etc.

6. Infection of congenital or acquired cysts

THE 'NORMAL' CHEST X-RAY

Faced in an exam. with a chest X-ray which at first sight appears
normal, consider the following possibilities:
  1. Small apical pneumothorax
  2. Hiatus hernia behind the heart
  3. Slight 'mitralisation' of the heart
  4. Skeletal defects, e.g. cervical rib
  5. Secondary deposits in ribs or clavicles
  6. Azygos lobe
  7. Unilateral mastectomy
  8. Gas under the diaphragm

CAUSES OF PNEUMOTHORAX

1. Traumatic

2. Iatrogenic
  (i) Thoracentesis, thoracic or cervical surgery
  (ii) Artificial pneumothorax
  (iii) Artificial ventilation

3. Spontaneous
   (i) *Localised air space disorder*
   Congenital bullae
   Localised emphysema
   Acquired cysts, etc.
   (ii) *Generalised emphysema*
   (iii) *Secondary to specific lung disease*
   Diffuse cystic disease
   e.g. congenital cysts, bronchiectasis, eosinophilic
   granuloma, tuberous sclerosis (epiloia)
   TB
   Silicosis
   Lung abscess
   Malignancy
   Hydatid cysts
   (iv) *Secondary to spontaneous mediastinal emphysema*
   Asthma, labour, straining at stool, etc.
   Rapid decompression of divers
   (v) *Associated with menstruation*
   ? Endometriosis

CAUSES OF PLEURAL EFFUSION

(A) *Transudate.* (Less than 25 g protein/litre. Implies a systemic cause).
   1. Cardiac failure
   2. Nephrotic syndrome
   3. Hepatic failure

(B) *Exudate.* (More than 25 g protein/litre. Implies a local cause).
   1. Pneumonia
   2. Malignancy (bronchial Ca., secondary Ca., lymphoma or mesothelioma)
   3. TB
   4. Pulmonary infarction
   5. Collagen-vascular disease (especially SLE)
   6. Subphrenic abscess
   7. Meig's syndrome (with ovarian fibroma)

FURTHER READING

Emerson P 1975 Medicine, 2nd series, 23: 1149
Turton C W G 1980 British Journal of Hospital Medicine 23: 239

CAUSES OF PULMONARY OEDEMA

1. **Increased capillary pressure**
     (i) Left heart failure
              Atrial, e.g. mitral stenosis
              Ventricular, e.g. hypertension or myocardial infarct
    (ii) Pulmonary venous obstruction
   (iii) Overload of i.v. fluid

2. **Increased capillary permeability**
     (i) Pneumonia (viral, bacterial)
    (ii) Inhaled toxins, e.g. chlorine, mustard gas
   (iii) Circulating toxins, e.g. paraquat, septicaemia, snake
              venoms, histamine
   (iv) Diffuse intravascular coagulation
    (v) Renal failure
   (vi) Radiation pneumonitis
  (vii) 'Shock-lung' (post-traumatic)

3. **Decreased plasma oncotic pressure**
    Hypo-albuminaemia

4. **Lymphatic obstruction**

5. **Unknown mechanism**
    High altitude
    Raised intra-cranial pressure
    Heroin overdose
    Pulmonary embolism, esp. fat
    Eclampsia

FURTHER READING

Flenley D C 1974 In: Ledingham J G G Advanced medicine, symposium 13.
   Pitman, London, p. 431

SHOCK LUNG
Acute respiratory insufficiency due to pulmonary oedema
progressing to interstitial fibrosis

Causes
1 'Shock' (p. 19)
2. Nonthoracic trauma
3. Sepsis
4. Overhydration
5. Disseminated intravascular coagulation

6. Massive transfusion
7. Fat embolism
8. Aspiration
9. CNS hypoxia
10. Oxygen toxicity
11. Drug overdose

FURTHER READING

Beyer A 1979 British Journal of Hospital Medicine 21: 248

COMPLICATIONS OF CA. BRONCHUS

A. Local effects
1. Bronchial obstruction
   collapse
   pneumonia
   abscess
   emphysema
2. SV Caval obstruction
3. Pulmonary artery or vein compression
4. Cervical sympathetic, recurrent laryngeal or phrenic invasion
5. Pleural effusion, empyema
6. Direct spread into mediastinum, chest wall, brachial plexus, etc.
7. Erosion of large vessel

B. Metastases
Hilar nodes, liver, cerebrum, adrenals, bone

C. Non-metastatic extra-pulmonary effects
1. Cachexia, anaemia etc.
2. Hypertrophic pulmonary osteoarthropathy and clubbing
3. Neuropathy or myopathy (p. 124)
4. Skin lesions (p. 185)
5. Ectopic humoral syndromes (p. 40)

N.B. *Polycythaemia* very rarely occurs with bronchial carcinoma, but may occur with renal carcinoma etc. (p. 158)

FURTHER READING

Rees Lesley 1978 Medicine, 3rd series, 10: 485
Riordan 1979 British Journal of Hospital Medicine 22: 120
Spiro S G 1979 Medicine, 3rd series, 23: 1201

Ectopic humoral syndromes

1. *ACTH and related peptides* (esp. oat cell Ca.)
   May account for 20% of cases of Cushing's syndrome
   Suspect the diagnosis in any patient with:
   (i) tumour + hypokalaemia
   (ii) Cushing's + high ACTH and cortisol
   (iii) Cushing's + hypokalaemia
   Confirm the diagnosis by:
   (i) Plasma ACTH: high
   (ii) 24 hr metapyrone test: usually no rise in ACTH in response to falling cortisol
   (iii) High dose dexamethasone test: usually no suppression
   (iv) ACTH measurement during selective venous catheterization
   (v) CAT scan may help, e.g. for thymic tumour
2. *Malignant hypercalcaemia* (esp. breast and lung Ca.)
   Possible mediators include:
   (i) Ectopic parathormone (rare)
   (ii) Prostaglandins
   (iii) Osteoclast-activating factor
   (iv) Vitamin D-like steroids
3. *Vasopressin* (esp. oat cell Ca.)
   Causes inappropriate diuresis
4. *Gonadotrophin* (esp. in tumours of testis, liver, stomach or pancreas)
   Causes precocious puberty in boys, and gynaecomastia in adult males.
5. *Calcitonin* (esp. oat cell Ca.)
   Occurs in about 50% of lung Ca. patients, but most are normocalcaemic
6. *Growth hormone or prolactin*
   Carcinoid may secrete GH-releasing factor
7. *Human placental lactogen*
   Causes gynaecomastia in males
8. *Thyrotrophin* (esp. in trophoblastic neoplasia, e.g. hydatidiform mole)
9. *Gastrointestinal hormones* (esp. VIP and somatostatin p. 73)
10. Serotin or catecholamines (carcinoid and phaeochromocytoma)
11. Pigmentation (hormone unknown)
12. Red cell aplasia or polycythaemia
13. Prostaglandin E_z
14. *Insulin*
    Doubtful entity, and hypoglycaemia may have other causes

FURTHER READING

Coombs R C 1982 British Journal of Hospital Medicine 27: 21
Rees Lesley 1981 In: Dawson A M, Compston N, Besser G M Recent
    advances in medicine—18. Churchill Livingstone, Edinburgh, p 261
Sherwood L M 1981 Medicine International 1: 279

HYPERTROPHIC OSTEOARTHROPATHY

A triad comprising
1. Clubbing
2. Periosteal new bone formation
3. Arthritis

CAUSES

1. **Thoracic**
    (i) Pulmonary neoplasm (Ca., mesothelioma)
    (ii) Chronic pulmonary suppuration
    (iii) Fibrosing alveolitis
    (iv) Mediastinal tumours, (p. 42)

2. **Cardio-vascular**
    (i) Bacterial endocarditis
    (ii) Cyanotic congenital heart disease
    (iii) Atrial myxoma
    (iv) Brachial arteriovenous fistula (unilateral)

3. **Extrathoracic lesions**
    (i) Gastro-enterological
       Cirrhosis (esp. biliary)
       Ulcerative colitis
       Crohn's disease
       Coeliac disease
    (ii) Thyrotoxicosis (thyroid acropachy)
    (iii) Rarely—Dysproteinaemia (esp. alpha chain disease)
               Pyelonephritis
               Syphilis
               Pregnancy

4. **Congenital** (*Pachydermoperiostosis*)
   The syndrome may be only partially expressed, e.g. congenital
   clubbing

Possible pathogenetic factors
1. Increased levels of growth hormone and oestrogens
2. Increased autonomic activity (stimulation of afferent tracts of the vagus)
3. Increased circulating levels of reduced ferritin

FURTHER READING

Katz W A 1977 Rheumatic disease, diagnosis and management. Lippincott, Philadelphia, p 676

Malignant tumours which metastasize to lung
1. Sarcomas
2. Bronchial Ca.
3. Breast Ca.
4. Renal Ca.
5. Thyroid Ca. } often clinically occult
6. Adrenal Ca.
7. Seminoma
8. Chorioepithelioma

Malignant tumours which metastasize to bone
1. Sarcomas
2. Bronchial Ca.
3. Breast Ca.
4. Prostatic Ca.
5. Renal Ca.
6. Thyroid Ca.
7. Neuroblastoma (in children)

MEDIASTINAL MASSES

Causes
1. *Lymphadenopathy*
   Lymphoma, sarcoidosis, infection (especially TB), carcinoma metastasis
2. *Aorta*
   Unfolding, aneurysm, coarctation
3. *Oesophagus*
   Corkscrew oesophagus (congenital elongation), megaoesophagus (achalasia), enterogenous cyst, neoplasm
4. *Retrosternal goitre*
5. *Cysts*
   Dermoid, teratoma, pericardial 'spring-water' cysts, hydatid, bronchial cyst
6. *Thymoma*

7. *Herniae*
   Hiatus hernia, diaphragmatic herniae, lung herniation
8. *Neurogenic*
   Neurilemmoma, neurofibroma, sympathetic ganglioneuroma,
   sympathetic neuroblastoma
9. *Miscellaneous rare causes*
   Cardiac aneurysm or tumour, mesothelioma, lipoma, etc.

FURTHER READING

Caplin M 1975 Medicine 2nd series, 23: 1148

Common sites of mediastinal tumours

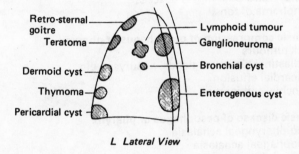

L Lateral View

Gastroenterology

CAUSES OF DYSPHAGIA

1. **Mouth and pharynx**
   Stomatitis and glossitis
   Tonsillitis
   Quinsy, retro-pharyngeal abscess
   Lymphoma of tonsil

2. **Extrinsic compression of oesophagus or pharynx**
   Neck tumours
   Mediastinal tumours, glands, aneurysm, etc.
   Pericardial effusion
   Bronchial carcinoma

3. **Intrinsic disease of oesophagus or pharynx**
   Crico-pharyngeal achalasia
   Oesophageal achalasia
   Plummer-Vinson syndrome
   (Fe def., glossitis, pharyngeal web and koilonychia)
   Pharyngeal pouch
   Inflammation, stricture, or neoplasm
   Systemic sclerosis
   Chagas' disease (trypanosomiasis)

4. **Foreign body**
   Within the lumen of oesophagus or pharynx

5. **CNS lesions**
   Bulbar and pseudo-bulbar palsy
   Myasthenia gravis
   Diphtheritic neuritis

6. **Psychological (globus hystericus)**

FURTHER READING

Atkinson M 1979 Medicine, 3rd series, 15: 759

CAUSES OF STOMATITIS

1. *Debilitation, smoking, alcoholism*
2. *Infection*
   (i) Viral
       Herpes simplex
       Herpangina
       Hand, foot and mouth disease
   (ii) Bacterial
       Pyorrhoea and alveolar abscess
       Vincent's angina, TB, Sy
   (iii) Fungal, especially Candida

3. *Associated with systemic disease*
   (i) Behcet's, Reiter's, Stevens-Johnson
   (ii) Leukaemia
   (iii) Neutropenia
   (iv) Fe deficiency
   (v) Vitamin deficiency
       B complex, including B_{12} and folate
   (vi) Cancrum oris (malnutrition, malaria etc.)

4. *Associated with skin disease*
   (i) Pemphigus vulgaris
   (ii) Benign pemphigoid of mucous membranes
   (iii) Lichen planus

5. *Stomatitis medicamentosa*
   (i) Cytotoxic drugs
   (ii) Bi, Hg, As, Au
   (iii) Antibiotics

6. *Aphthous ulcers*

7. *Leukoplakia*

8. *Neoplasm*

9. *Allergy*
e.g. dentures and dental medicaments

10. *Caustics and trauma*
e.g. cheek-biting and dentures

Systemic causes of gingival swelling
1. Pregnancy and oral contraceptives
2. Leukaemia (especially monocytic)
3. Phenytoin
4. Scurvy
5. Heavy metals (especially Hg and As)

CAUSES OF VOMITING

1. Feeding upsets (in infancy) and dietary indiscretions

2. GI irritation
   Poisons
   Gastric ulcer
   Gastritis
   Enteritis

3. Obstruction
   Atresia
   Stricture (including malignancy) or stenosis
   Intussusception
   Volvulus
   Strangulated hernia
   Paralytic ileus

4. Acute intra-abdominal inflammation
   Hepatitis
   Pancreatitis
   Appendicitis
   Pyelonephritis
   Cholecystitis

5. Metabolic and endocrine
   Diabetic precoma
   Pregnancy
   Uraemia
   Hypoadrenalism

6. CNS
   Psychogenic
   Severe pain
   Drugs
   Migraine
   Motion sickness
   Meningitis
   Menière's, labyrinthitis
   Raised intra-cranial pressure

7. **Miscellaneous**
   Acute dilatation of stomach
   Cyclical vomiting
   Radiation sickness
   Pertussis, etc.

CAUSES OF PAROTID GLAND ENLARGEMENT

1. **Infections**
   (i) Viral (mumps, cytomegalic inclusion disease)
   (ii) Bacterial, especially in dehydrated patients

2. **Neoplasia**

3. **Duct blockage**
   e.g. by calculus

4. **Systemic disease**
   (i) Sjögren's syndrome
   (ii) Sarcoidosis
   (iii) Drugs (Iodides, thiouracil, phenylbutazone, lead)
   (iv) Cirrhosis
   (v) Cystic fibrosis
   (vi) Rarely—hyperlipidaemia, malnutrition or vitamin deficiency, pregnancy, diabetes mellitus

FURTHER READING

Katz W A 1977 Rheumatic disease, diagnosis and management. Lippincott, Philadelphia, p 211

CAUSES OF CONSTIPATION

ACUTE

1. *Ileus*
2. *Obstruction*
3. *'Simple' constipation* due to acute illness, hospital admission, travel, dehydration, low food intake, etc.
4. *Painful ano-rectal disease*, e.g. fissure

(contd)

CHRONIC

1. Disordered intestinal motility

    (i) *Small faecal residue*, e.g. low fibre diet, dehydration
    (ii) *Over-use of purgatives*
    (iii) *Idiopathic bowel disorder*
        Irritable bowel syndrome (spastic colon)
        Idiopathic slow transit
        Idiopathic megabowel
    (iv) *Secondary to inflammatory bowel disease*
        e.g. diverticulitis,
        ulcerative colitis
    (v) *Metabolic*
        Early pregnancy
        Hypothyroidism
        Hypercalcaemia
        Hypokalaemia
        Acute intermittent porphyria
        Lead poisoning
    (vi) *Drugs*
        Opiate derivatives
        Ganglion-blockers
        Anticholinergics
        Aluminium hydroxide
        Cholestyramine
        Iron salts
    (vii) *Neuro-muscular disease*
        Spinal cord lesions
        Autonomic neuropathy
        Chagas' disease (toxic destruction of myenteric
        neurones)
        Systemic sclerosis (gut muscle degeneration)
        Hirschsprung's disease (genetic aganglionosis)
    (viii) *Psychiatric*
        Depression, psychosis, anorexia nervosa, mental
        subnormality

2. Obstruction

Stricture, tumour, etc.

3. Rectal dyschezia (habitual neglect of call to stool)

FURTHER READING

Hinton J M 1972 In: Avery-Jones F, Godding E W (eds) Management of
constipation. Blackwell, Oxford, p 79

CAUSES OF DIARRHOEA

ACUTE

1. **Dietary indiscretion**, e.g. unripe fruit

2. **Food poisoning**
   Animal
   Plant
   Bacterial (endotoxin or exotoxin)
   Chemical

3. **Gastro-intestinal infection**
   Viral
   Bacterial
   Protozoal
   Helminthic

4. **Allergy**

5. **Psychogenic** (esp. anxiety)

CHRONIC

1. **Gastric**
   Gastrectomy
   Vagotomy
   Linitis plastica
   Pernicious anaemia

2. **Intestinal**
   Ulcerative colitis
   Crohn's disease
   Diverticular disease
   Neoplasm, etc.

3. **Malabsorption** (p. 50)

4. **Metabolic**
   Thyrotoxicosis
   Medullary carcinoma of thyroid
   Pellagra
   Gut endocrine tumours (p. 73)

5. **Drugs**
   e.g. purgatives

6. **Autonomic neuropathy**
   e.g. diabetes

7. **Spurious diarrhoea**
   (due to faecal impaction)

CAUSES OF MALABSORPTION

1. **Inadequate digestion**
   Gastric or intestinal resection
   Bile salt deficiency
   Pancreatic insufficiency (especially fibrocystic disease)
   Disorders of enterocyte brush border
      (i) Disaccharidase deficiency
      (ii) Enterokinase deficiency

2. **Parasites**
   Tapeworms
   Giardiasis, Strongyloides stercoralis, Diphyllobothrium latum

3. **Change in intestinal bacterial flora** (p. 51)

4. **Intestinal hurry or fistulae**

5. **Enterocyte damage**
   Coeliac disease (Gluten intolerance)
   Cow's milk intolerance
   Soya flour intolerance
   Tropical sprue

6. **Infiltrative disorders**
   Crohn's disease
   Whipple's disease
   Lymphoma or leukaemia
   TB
   Systemic sclerosis
   Systemic mastocytosis
   Alpha-chain disease
   Amyloidosis

7. **Metabolic abnormality**
   Hartnup disease (malabsorption of neutral amino acids)
   Cystinuria (malabsortion of dibasic amino acids)
   Abetalipoproteinaemia
   Carcinoid
   Carcinomatous enteropathy
   Dermatogenic enteropathy (extensive eczema or psoriasis)

8. **Endocrine**
   Addison's hypoadrenalism
   Hypoparathyroidism
   Hyperthyroidism
   Medullary carcinoma of thyroid
   Zollinger-Ellison syndrome
   Werner-Morrison syndrome   (p. 73)
   Diabetes mellitus

9. **Vascular**
   Mesenteric arterial insufficiency
   Chronic venous congestion
   Lymphangiectasia

10. **Drugs**
    Liquid paraffin
    Neomycin, colchicine, cholestyramine etc.

11. **Radiation enteritis**

FURTHER READING

Losowsky M S 1979 Medicine, 3rd series 16: 790

CAUSES OF ABNORMAL GUT FLORA

1. **Abnormalities of gastric function**
   (i) Polya partial gastrectomy——Afferent loop syndrome
   (ii) Malfunctioning gastro-jejunostomy
   (iii) Pernicious anaemia

2. **Stasis**
   (i) Surgical blind loops
   (ii) Strictures
   (iii) Adhesions
   (iv) Small intestinal diverticulosis
   (v) Abnormal motility
   Systemic sclerosis
   Autonomic neuropathy
   Vagotomy
   Ganglion blocking agents
   (vi) Partial biliary obstruction with cholangitis

3. **Free communications between large and small bowel**
   (i) Gastrocolic fistula
   (ii) Enterocolic fistula
   (iii) Massive intestinal resection

FURTHER READING

Tabaqchali S 1973 In: Truelove S C, Jewell D P (eds) Topics in
  gastroenterology, vol 1, Blackwell, Oxford, p 156

CAUSES OF HEPATOMEGALY

1. **Raised venous pressure**
   Congestive cardiac failure
   Constrictive pericarditis
   Tricuspid stenosis
   Hepatic vein obstruction (Budd-Chiari)

2. **Degenerative**
   Fatty infiltration and early cirrhosis (esp. alcoholic)
   Reye's syndrome

3. **Myeloproliferative** (p. 89)

4. **Neoplastic**
   Primary (hepatoma, etc)
   Metastases
   Lymphoma

5. **Infective**
   Viral—Infective and serum hepatitis
           Infectious mononucleosis
   Bacterial—Hepatic abscess
             TB, Syphilis
             Brucellosis
             Weil's disease
   Protozoal—Amoebic abscess
             Malaria
             Toxoplasmosis
             Kala-azar
   Parasitic—Hydatid cyst

6. **Storage disorders**
   Amyloidosis
   Gaucher's
   Niemann-Pick's
   Histiocytosis X
   Glycogen storage disease
   Haemochromatosis
   Hurler's (gargoylism)

7. **Biliary obstruction**

8. **Congenital**
   Riedel's lobe (palpable, but not enlarged)
   Polycystic disease
   Congenital hepatic fibrosis

Causes of a hard knobbly liver

1. Carcinoma metastases
2. Cirrhosis with hepatoma
3. Polycystic liver
4. Hydatid cysts
5. Hepar lobatum (syphilis)

Causes of hepato-splenomegaly

1. Infective, e.g. Infectious mononucleosis
2. Myeloproliferative, e.g. Myelofibrosis, chronic myeloid leukaemia
3. Some causes of portal hypertension, e.g. Budd-Chiari syndrome
4. Reticuloses
5. Storage diseases, e.g. Gaucher's disease, amyloidosis
6. Anaemia, e.g. PA, sickle-cell anaemia in children

CAUSES OF CIRRHOSIS

1. **Infection**
     (i) Viral hepatitis A and B
    (ii) ? Other viruses
   (iii) Congenital syphilis

2. **Toxins**
     (i) Alcohol
    (ii) Drugs e.g. methyldopa

3. **Prolonged cholestasis**
   e.g. biliary stricture

4. **Immunological**
     (i) Primary biliary (Hanot's)
    (ii) Active chronic hepatitis

5. **Metabolic**
     (i) Haemochromatosis
    (ii) Hepato-lenticular degeneration (Wilson's)
   (iii) Galactosaemia
    (iv) Fructosaemia
     (v) Glycogen storage disease
    (vi) Tyrosinosis
   (vii) Alpha-1 antitrypsin deficiency

(contd)

6. Venous stasis
    (i) Prolonged congestive cardiac failure
    (ii) Hepatic vein occlusion

7. Miscellaneous
    (i) Cystic fibrosis
    (ii) Hereditary haemorrhagic telangiectasia (Osler's)
    (iii) Sickle-cell disease
    (iv) Jejuno-ileal bypass (for obesity)

8. Idiopathic

FURTHER READING

Brunt P W 1975 Medicine 2nd series 21: 991

Complications of chronic biliary obstruction
1. Liver cell dysfunction
2. Acute oliguric renal failure (especially in the elderly)
3. Metabolic bone disease (osteomalacia or osteoporosis) and hyperpara thyroidism
4. Vitamin K deficiency
5. Hyperlipidaemia
6. Infection of biliary tree, and septicaemia
7. Pigmentation
8. Pruritus
9. Weight loss due to malabsorption

FURTHER READING

Read A E 1979 Medicine, 3rd series, 17: 850

Disorders associated with primary biliary cirrhosis
1. Systemic sclerosis (including CRST syndrome)
2. Sjogren's syndrome, rheumatoid disease or SLE
3. Thyroiditis
4. Renal tubular acidosis
5. Lichen planus

FURTHER READING

Losowsky M 1979 Medicine, 3rd series, 17: 884

Causes of intra-hepatic cholestasis

In children
Biliary atresia
Neonatal (giant cell) hepatitis
Galectosaemia
Mucoviscidosis
α1-anti-trypsin deficiency
Viral hepatitis
Byler disease (a genetic bile duct disorder)

In adults
Drugs (e.g. methyl testosterone, synthetic oestrogens, phenothiazines)
Viral hepatitis
Primary biliary cirrhosis
Alcohol
Pregnancy
Inflammatory bowel disease
Cirrhosis
Idiopathic

FURTHER READING

Read A E 1979 British Journal of Hospital Medicine 21: 490

PORTAL HYPERTENSION

CAUSES

1. **Extra-hepatic presinusoidal (Portal vein thrombosis)**
   Umbilical sepsis, exchange transfusion in neonates
   Suppurative pylephlebitis
   Portal lymphadenopathy (Ca. metastasis, lymphoma, etc)
   Clotting diathesis e.g. polycythaemia

2. **Intra-hepatic presinusoidal**
   Schistosomiasis
   Sarcoid, Hodgkin's, leukaemic infiltrates
   Congenital hepatic fibrosis

3. **Intra-hepatic postsinusoidal**
   Cirrhosis
   Veno-occlusive disease (Jamaican bush-tea)

(contd)

4. Extra-hepatic postsinusoidal
Hepatic vein obstruction (Budd-Chiari)
Constrictive pericarditis, etc.

When obstruction is presinusoidal, hepatic function is relatively unimpaired, and bleeding from varices does not cause liver failure

IDEAL CRITERIA FOR PORTA-CAVAL SHUNT

1. Age under 40
2. Portal vein patent
3. Se Bilirubin < 25 μmol/l, Se Albumin > 30 g/l
4. No ascites
5. No previous episodes of precoma
6. Good nutrition
7. High I.Q. not essential for patient's occupation

Complications of porta-caval shunts
1. Operative risks
2. Encephalopathy and myelopathy
3. Hyperbilirubinaemia
4. Gastric hyperacidity
5. Haemochromatosis

FURTHER READING

Shields R 1979 Medicine, 3rd series, 17: 876

HEPATIC ENCEPHALOPATHY

Cerebral dysfunction which can complicate all forms of liver disease and which particularly affects consciousness. The mean EEG frequency is slowed, nitrogenous substances are retained in the brain and giant astrocytes proliferate.

Clinical types of hepatic encephalopathy
1. *Chronic portasystemic encephalopathy*
2. *Cirrhosis with a precipitant*
   e.g.
   Diuresis
   Haemorrhage
   Paracentesis abdominis
   Diarrhoea and vomiting
   Surgery
   Alcohol
   Sedatives
   Infections

3. *Acute liver failure*
   e.g. due to
   Viral hepatitis
   Alcoholic hepatitis
   Drug reactions
   Paracetamol overdose

Factors affecting hepatic encephalopathy
1. Portasystemic collaterals
   (i) Extrahepatic e.g. varices, shunt
   (ii) Intrahepatic e.g. around cirrhotic nodules
2. Nitrogenous content of intestines
3. Bacterial action on colonic contents
4. Liver cell function

FURTHER READING

Sherlock Sheila 1977 British Journal of Hospital Medicine 17: 144.
Silk D B A 1979 British Journal of Hospital Medicine 22: 437

PATTERNS OF HEPATOCYTE INJURY

1. **Direct**
   Characterized by mitochondrial damage, central necrosis and, usually, fatty change
   (i) Alcohol
       Obesity ⎫ Predominantly mitochondrial
       Diabetes mellitus ⎬ damage
       Wilson's disease ⎭
   (ii) Reye's syndrome
        Tetracycline toxicity ⎫ Damage to mitochondria and
        Fatty liver of pregnancy ⎬ ribosomes
        Cytotoxic drugs ⎭
   (iii) Metabolite-related, e.g. isoniazid is converted to an acylating agent
   (iv) Anoxia, e.g. 'shock' or hepatic venous obstruction
   (v) Heavy-metal escape from lysosomes, e.g. haemochromatosis

2. **Immunological**
   Characterized by damage to cell membranes, piecemeal necrosis of periportal hepatocytes and mononuclear infiltrates
   (i) Chronic active hepatitis
   (ii) Primary biliary cirrhosis
   (iii) Drug reactions, e.g. halothane

(*contd*)

3. Cholestatic
Characterized by retention of bile in liver cells and canaliculi, with secondary effects on other organelles
  (i) Extrahepatic, e.g. due to stones in bile duct
  (ii) Intrahepatic, e.g. due to sex hormones

FURTHER READING

Sheila Sherlock 1982 Lancet i: 782

HEPATITIS

CLINICAL VARIANTS

Acute
1. Anicteric hepatitis
2. Classical acute hepatitis
3. Cholestatic hepatitis
4. Relapsing hepatitis
5. Fulminant hepatitis
6. Subacute hepatic necrosis

Chronic sequelae
1. Chronic persistent hepatitis
2. Active chronic hepatitis (q.v.)
3. Asymptomatic carrier state

FURTHER READING

Sherlock S 1975 In: Last A F (ed) Advanced medicine, symposium II. Pitman London, p 72
Woolf I., Williams R 1977 British Journal of Hospital Medicine 17: 117

ACTIVE CHRONIC HEPATITIS (formerly called 'lupoid hepatitis')

A chronic disease, predominantly affecting the liver, with continuing damage to hepatocytes and with evidence of abnormal immunological activity.

Possible aetiological factors
1. Viral hepatitis
2. Drugs—Oxyphenisatin, methyldopa, isoniazid
3. Other chronic liver disease, especially alcoholic
4. Alpha$_1$—antitrypsin deficiency

Antibody reactions	% Positive cases			
	Active chronic hepatitis	Primary biliary cirrhosis	SLE	Control population
Anti-nuclear factor	65	40	>95	<5
Anti-mitochondrial	10	90	10	<1
Anti-smooth muscle	70	5	<1	3
Anti-glomerular	50	<1	<1	<1

FURTHER READING

Joske R A 1975 In: Read A E (ed) Modern trends in gastroenterology, vol 5. Butterworth, London, p 418
Sherlock S 1979 Medicine, 3rd series, 18: 909

LIVER TUMOURS

CAUSES OF PRIMARY LIVER TUMOURS

Hepatocellular Ca.
1. Cirrhosis
2. Toxins
   (i) Aflatoxin (a metabolite of a mould which grows on rice and peanuts)
   (ii) Nitrosamines
3. Anabolic androgens
4. ? Poor nutrition

Cholangiocarcinoma
1. Parasitic infestation of biliary tree
   (i) Liver fluke—Clonorchis sinensis
   (ii) Schistosomiasis

Angiosarcoma
1. Previous 'Thorotrast' injection (for radiography)
2. Arsenic
3. Vinyl chloride monomer

FURTHER READING

Kew M C 1979 Medicine, 3rd series, 17: 864
Terblanche J 1977 British Journal of Hospital Medicine 17: 103

ALPHA-FETOPROTEIN (AFP)

Occurs in plasma in:
1. Normal fetus
2. Elevated maternal AFP may indicate fetal neural-tube defect, twin pregnancy, intrauterine death, threatened abortion or subsequent low birth-weight
3. Hepatoma (in 90%)
4. Infective hepatitis, cirrhosis or liver metastases
5. Occasionally in primary Ca. of stomach, ovary or testis

Occurs in increased conc. in amniotic fluid in:
1. Anencephaly
2. Open spina bifida
3. Omphalocoele
4. Bowel atresia
5. Turner syndrome
6. Congenital nephrosis
7. Intra-uterine death

FURTHER READING

Harper P S 1976 In: Peters D K (ed) Advanced medicine, symposium 12.
  Pitman, London, p 457
Kew M C 1975 In: Read A E (ed) Modern trends in gastroenterology, vol 5.
  Butterworth, London, p 91

SOME 'METABOLIC' EFFECTS OF LIVER CELL CARCINOMA

1. Hypoglycaemia
2. Hypercalcaemia
3. Hyperlipidaemia
4. Hypertrophic pulmonary osteoarthropathy
5. Erythrocytosis
6. Dysfibrinogenaemia
7. Porphyria cutanea tarda
8. Carcinoid syndrome
9. Sexual precocity

FURTHER READING

Murray-Lyon I M 1975 Medicine, 2nd series, 21: 1004

HAEMOCHROMATOSIS

Haemosiderosis implies a pathological increase in tissue iron levels, but is not necessarily accompanied by cell damage

Haemochromatosis implies increased tissue iron with accompanying cell damage

Causes of haemochromatosis
1. *Primary* (dominant with incomplete penetrance)
2. *Secondary*
    (i) Multiple blood transfusions
    (ii) Inability to utilise iron
        a. Sideroblastic anaemia
        b. Thalassaemia
        c. Sickle-cell anaemia
    (iii) Increased iron ingestion (e.g. Kaffir beer made in iron cooking pots)
    (iv) Liver disease, especially due to alcohol
    (v) Porta-caval shunt
    (vi) Porphyria cutanea tarda
    (vii) Xanthinuria
    (viii) Congenital transferrin deficiency

FURTHER READING

Dymock I W 1975 In: Read A E (ed) Modern trends in gastroenterology, vol 5. Butterworth, London, p 345
Brown E B 1981 Advances in internal medicine, vol 26 Year Book Medical Publishers, Chicago, p 159–178

LIVER DISEASE DUE TO DRUGS OR CHEMICALS

1. *Hepatic necrosis due to toxins*
    Halogenated hydrocarbons
    Heavy metals
    Iron or paracetamol overdose
2. *Hepatitis*
    Monoamine oxidase inhibitors
    Antidepressants
    Antirheumatic drugs
    Anticonvulsants
3. *Cholestasis*
    (i) Hypersensitivity, e.g. chlorpromazine
    (ii) Steroid-cholestasis, e.g. 17-methyltestosterone
4. *Generalised hypersensitivity*, e.g. antibiotics
5. *Hepatic vein occlusion*
    Plant toxins ('bush teas')
    Oral contraceptives

(contd)

6. *Fibrosis or cirrhosis*
   Cytotoxins, especially methotrexate
7. *Interference with normal bilirubin pathway* (normal liver histology)
   (i) Haemolysis, e.g. methyldopa
   (ii) Decreased uptake, e.g. Filix mas
   (iii) Conjugation defect, e.g. novobiocin
   (iv) Competition with bilirubin, e.g. X-ray contrast media
   (v) Protein-binding release, e.g. salicylates
8. *Hepatic hyperplasia, adenoma or carcinoma*
   Anabolic and androgenic steroids
   Oral contraceptives
   Nitrosamines
9. *Fibrosis or angiosarcoma*
   Arsenic
   Thorotrast
   Vinyl chloride

FURTHER READING

Davis M 1980 British Journal of Hospital Medicine 24: 17
Sherlock Sheila 1975 Medicine, 2nd series, 21: 979

MECHANISMS OF DRUG INTERACTIONS

A. PHARMACEUTICAL

e.g. drug interacting with incompatible infusion fluid

B. PHARMACOKINETIC

1. *Absorption*
   e.g. (i) noradrenaline and local anaesthetics
        (ii) liquid paraffin and fat-soluble drugs
        (iii) chelating agents such as cholestyramine
2. *Elimination*
   (i) Hepatic metabolism, e.g. enzyme stimulation by phenobarbitone
   (ii) Renal excretion, e.g. salicylates reduce tubular secretion of methotrexate
3. *Distribution*
   e.g. (i) Drugs bound by protein displace each other (sulphonamides, warfarin, tolbutamide, phenylbutazone, etc.)
        (ii) Quinidine displaces digoxin from tissues

C. PHARMACODYNAMIC

1. *Competition at receptor sites*
   e.g. (i) nalorphine and morphine
   (ii) acetylcholine and anticholinergics
2. *'Physiological' interactions*
   (i) Antagonists, e.g. histamine and adrenaline
   (ii) Additives, e.g. barbiturates and alcohol
   (iii) Potentiators, e.g. digitalis and diuretics (hypokalaemia)

FURTHER READING

Dollery C T 1972 In: Neale G (ed) Advanced medicine, symposium 8.
   Pitman, London, p 185
Routledge P A, Sand D G 1981 In: Dawson A M, Compston N, Besser G
M (eds) Recent advances in medicine—18. Churchill Livingstone,
   Edinburgh, p 39

FAMILIAL NON-HAEMOLYTIC JAUNDICE

Unconjugated
1. *Gilbert's*
   Decreased uptake of bilirubin by liver cell
   Mild intermittent jaundice
2. *Primary 'shunt' hyperbilirubinaemia*
   Increased production of bilirubin in marrow
   Very rare
3. *Crigler-Najjar*
   Hepatic glucuronyl-transferase deficiency
   Poor prognosis. Extremely rare
4. *Familial neonatal hyperbilirubinaemia*
   Glucuronyl-transferase inhibitor in serum
5. *Breast milk jaundice*
   Glucuronyl-transferase inhibitor in breast milk

Conjugated
1. *Dubin-Johnson*
   Mild intermittent jaundice
   Brown pigment in liver cells
   Characteristic BSP test with secondary rise at 2 hr due to
   re-entry of conjugated bilirubin into blood
2. *Rotor*
   Similar but without hepatic pigmentation
3. *Summerskill and Walshe*
   Recurrent cholestasis of unknown case

FURTHER READING

Israel J B, Arias I M 1976 Advances in Internal Medicine 21: 77

CAUSES OF HYPOCHLORHYDRIA

1. Pernicious anaemia
2. Gastric ulcer
3. Gastric carcinoma
4. Gastric polyposis
5. Subtotal gastrectomy
6. Iron deficiency
7. Pregnancy
8. Atrophic gastritis
9. Old age of debility
10. Vitamin deficiency (pellagra)
11. Radiation

CAUSES OF HAEMATEMESIS

1. Peptic ulcer
2. Oesophageal varices
3. Erosive gastritis (aspirin, alcohol, etc.)
4. Hiatus hernia
5. Erosive oesophagitis
6. Mallory-Weiss syndrome (Oesophageal tear)
7. Swallowed blood
8. Blood dyscrasia
9. Gastric neoplasm
10. Haemorrhagic telangiectasia (Osler-Weber-Rendu)
11. Pseudoxanthoma elasticum
12. Ehlers-Danlos syndrome (Cutis hyperelastica)

PEPTIC ULCER

Indications for surgical treatment of peptic ulcer
1. Perforation
2. Continuous or intermittent bleeding
3. Pyloric stenosis
4. Suspicion of malignancy, e.g. ulcer on greater curve, or positive cytology
5. Failure of medical treatment
6. Economic considerations and expediency
7. Serious persistent hour-glass deformity
8. Combined GU and DU
9. Very large ulcers
10. Gastric ulcer in patient over 60 with a short history

Side effects of vagotomy
1. Atony of stomach with dilatation
2. Belching and 'bilious' feeling
3. Abdominal distension
4. Diarrhoea
5. Cardiospasm

Medical complications of gastrectomy
1. Calorie deficiency
2. Stomal ulcer
3. 'Dumping syndrome'
4. Bilious vomiting, distension
5. Post-prandial diarrhoea
6. Malabsorption
7. Anaemia (deficiency of Fe, B_{12} or folate)
8. Osteomalacia
9. Hypoanabolic hypoproteinaemia
10. Increased risk of carcinoma in gastric remnant
11. Recrudescence of pulmonary TB

FURTHER READING

Langman M, Alexander-Williams J 1979 Medicine, 3rd series, 15: 769

CAUSES OF CALCIFICATION ON ABDOMINAL X-RAY
1. Phleboliths
2. Calcified lymph nodes
3. Calculi (renal, gall-bladder, prostatic)
4. Calcified pancreas, adrenal, liver, kidney, aorta, psoas muscle, costal cartilage, etc.
5. Calcified tumour—dermoid, fibroid, etc.
6. Calcification in abdominal wall, e.g. cysticerci
7. Faecolith
8. Fetus

FURTHER READING

Armstrong P 1976 British Journal of Hospital Medicine 15: 597

CAUSES OF A MASS IN R. ILIAC FOSSA
1. Appendix abscess
2. Carcinoma caecum
3. Crohn's disease
4. Ileocaecal TB
5. Intussusception
6. Ovarian tumour, tubal pregnancy, etc.
7. Ectopic kidney
8. Actinomycosis
9. Carcinoid
10. Amoebiasis
11. Schistosomiasis

CAUSES OF ACUTE PANCREATITIS

1. **Biliary tract disease, including gall-stones**
2. **Alcohol**
3. **Idiopathic**
4. **Metabolic**
    (i)   Hyperparathyroidism
    (ii) Hypercalcaemia
    (iii) Hyperlipidaemia
    (iv) Pregnancy and post-partum
5. **Trauma or surgery**
6. **Congenital defects**
    e.g. obstructed pancreatic duct
7. **Drugs**
    (i)   Morphine
    (i)   Steroids
    (iii) Thiazide diuretics
8. **Viral**
    (i)   Mumps
    (ii) Infectious hepatitis
    (iii) Infectious mononucleosis
9. **Parasitic**
    (i)   Ascaris lumbricoides
    (ii) Clonorchis sinensis
10. **Vascular disease**
11. **Carcinoma of pancreas**
12. **Hypothermia**

FURTHER READING

Howat H T, Sarles H 1979 The exocrine pancreas. W B Saunders, London
Bouchier I 1979 Medicine, 3rd series, 18: 938

CAUSES OF PROTEIN-LOSING GASTROENTEROPATHY

1. Giant gastric rugae (Ménétrier's)
2. Ulcerative colitis, Crohn's disease
3. Sprue
4. Intestinal lipodystrophy (Whipple's)
5. Malignancy, esp. gastric Ca.
6. Intestinal lymphangiectasia
7. Constrictive pericarditis, congestive cardiac failure
8. Hypogammaglobulinaemia
9. Erythroderma
10. 'Allergic gastroenteropathy' (? milk allergy)

MEDICAL CAUSES OF ACUTE ABDOMINAL PAIN

Some uncommon causes
1. Gastric dilatation, esp. in diabetic ketosis
2. Ischaemic bowel (q.v.)
3. Migraine
4. Epilepsy
5. Lead poisoning
6. Tabes dorsalis
7. Acute intermittent porphyria
8. Addison's disease
9. Haemochromatosis
10. Haemolytic crisis (especially sickle-cell anaemia)
11. Henoch-Schönlein purpura
12. Hepatoma
13. Hypercalcaemia
14. Uraemia
15. Intestinal parasites

Acute small bowel ischaemia

Causes
1. Thrombosis of superior mesenteric artery (e.g. due to atheroma, polycythaemia or oestrogens)
2. Embolism of superior mesenteric artery (e.g. secondary to myocardial infarct)
3. Low-flow non-occlusive states
   (i) Narrowing of superior mesenteric artery trunk
   (ii) Splanchnic vasoconstriction (e.g. digoxin overdose)
   (iii) Low cardiac output
   (iv) Haemoconcentration

Classical features
   (i) Abrupt onset of severe abdominal pain
   (ii) Paradoxical absence of abdominal signs
   (iii) Rapid onset of hypovolaemic shock

Chronic small bowel ischaemia
Defined as a reduction of the post-prandial intestinal blood flow sufficient to cause abdominal pain
Cause: Narrowing of at least 2 of the 3 visceral branches of the aorta (coeliac axis, superior mesenteric or inferior mesenteric)

Classical features
1. Severe upper abdominal colicky pain soon after eating, often with borborygmi
2. Weight loss due to 'food fear'
3. Initial constipation, progressing to malabsorption
4. Epigastric bruit conducted to right iliac fossa

FURTHER READING

Marcuson R 1979 Medicine, 3rd series, 15: 766

COMPLICATIONS AND ASSOCIATIONS OF ULCERATIVE COLITIS

1. **Nutritional deficiencies**

   Anaemia   Hypokalaemia
   Vitamin deficiency   Hypoproteinaemia
   Dehydration

2. **Colonic**

   Acute toxic dilatation   Confluent crypt abscesses
   Perforation   Carcinoma
   Massive bleeding   Stricture (in 10%, but rarely
                              causes symptoms)

3. **Anal**

   Haemorrhoids   Anal fistula
   Anal fissure   Perianal abscess

4. **Ectodermal**

   Aphthous ulcers   Erythema multiforme
   Clubbing   Pyoderma gangrenosum
   Erythema nodosum

5. **Arthritis**

   Polyarthritis   Ankylosing spondylitis
   Sacro-iliitis

6. **Ocular**

   Uveitis   Retinitis
   Episcleritis   Retrobulbar neuritis
   Keratitis

7. Hepatic

Fatty infiltration	Cirrhosis and chronic active
Granulomata	hepatitis
Focal necrosis	Pericholangitis
Abscess (portal	Sclerosing cholangitis
bacteriaemia)	Rarely, biliary tract carcinoma

8. Renal

Pyelonephritis   Calculi

9. Thrombo-phlebitis

10. Iatrogenic (drugs, transfusions, surgery, etc.)

FURTHER READING

Jewell D, Mee A 1979 Medicine, 3rd series, 16: 802

COMPLICATIONS OF CROHN'S DISEASE

1. Intestinal
Small bowel obstruction
Fistulae, esp. into bladder, or vagina
Perforation
Suppuration and abscess formation
Stricture
Bleeding (usually slow, but may be massive)

2. Ectodermal
Aphthous ulcers
Clubbing
Erythema nodosum
Erythema multiforme
Pyoderma gangrenosum
Crohn's disease of mouth or skin (peri-anal or peri-ileostomy)
Ectopic Crohn's of skin not contiguous to intestinal mucosa

3. Nutritional deficiencies (as for UC, p. 68)
Due to
(i) Decreased food intake
(ii) Malabsorption—reduction in absorptive surface
        disaccharidase deficiency
        altered intestinal flora
        intestinal hurry
(iii) Loss of blood or protein into bowel
(iv) Increased metabolic requirement

4. Arthritis

5. Ocular } as for U.C. (p. 68)

6. Renal

7. Amyloidosis is commoner in Crohn's than in U.C.

8. Hepatic complications are less common in Crohn's than in U.C., but cholesterol gallstones occur

FURTHER READING

Dyer N 1975 Medicine, 2nd series, 19: 898
Sleisenger M H, Fordtran J S 1973 Gastrointestinal disease. Saunders, Philadelphia, p 896

CAUSES OF MULTIPLE INTESTINAL POLYPS

1. Neoplastic
    (i) Familial adenomatous polyposis coli
          Autosomal dominant
          Presents with diarrhoea
          Malignancy invariably develops
    Some patients have Gardner's syndrome (epidermoid cysts, osteomas, dentigerous cysts, lipomas, dermatofibromas)

2. Hamartomatous
    (i) 'Juvenile' polyposis coli
          Presents with prolapse or bleeding P.R.
          Not pre-malignant
    (ii) Peutz-Jeghers
          Peri-orificial lentiginosis with polyps mainly in small intestine
          Presents with anaemia or intussusception
          Very rarely associated with Ca. stomach or colon

3. Inflammatory
    Pseudo-polyposis
    Secondary to ulcerative colitis or colonic Crohn's

4. Cronkhite-Canada syndrome
    Generalised G.I. polyposis with alopecia, pigmentation and nail dystrophy. Very rare

FURTHER READING

Hawley P R 1979 Medicine, 3rd series, 16: 814.

COMPLICATIONS OF PARENTERAL NUTRITION

1. Complications of central-vein catheterization
    (i) Perforation of heart or blood vessel
   (ii) Thrombosis of vessel
  (iii) Air embolism
   (iv) Pneumothorax
    (v) Febrile reactions to pyrogens in tubing
   (vi) Infections, especially yeast or fungal
  (vii) Damage to thoracic duct or brachial plexus

2. Reactions to nutrients or lack of nutrients
     (i) Allergic reaction
    (ii) Hyperosmolar syndrome with dehydration
   (iii) Hypoglycaemia on rapid cessation of glucose infusion
   (iv) Hyperchloraemic or lactic acidosis
    (v) Hypophosphataemia
   (vi) Fluid overload and electrolyte inbalance
  (vii) Deficiency states
 (viii) Acne conglobata

FURTHER READING

Law D H 1972 Advances in Internal Medicine 18: 389
Powell-Tuck J 1979 Medicine, 3rd series, 16: 825.

CARCINO-EMBRYONIC ANTIGEN (CEA)

Occurs in plasma in:
1. Malignancy
   (i) endodermal adenocarcinoma (i.e. GI tract)
  (ii) bronchus, breast, neuroblastoma, female reproductive tract
     Higher values occur with poorly differentiated tumours, and
     after metastasis (over 100 ng/ml)
2. Non-neoplastic disease of pancreas, liver or colon

FURTHER READING

Brostoff J, Walker G 1975 In: Taylor G (ed) Immunology in medical practice.
  Saunders, London, p 196

GUT HORMONES (the 'diffuse endocrine' system)

Functions	Major hormones responsible
Control of secretions and motility of stomach and intestine	Motilin, gastrin, VIP, glucagon-like peptide
Control of gallbladder function	Cholecystokinin and pancreatic peptide
Control of exocrine pancreas	Secretin, cholecystokinin, VIP and pancreatic peptide
Control of pancreatic islet secretion	Gastric inhibitory polypeptide
Metabolism of fat, protein and carbohydrate	Insulin, glucagon, somatostatin
Neurotransmitter functions	Substance P, VIP and enkephalins

DISTRIBUTION OF PEPTIDES IN THE GASTROINTESTINAL TRACT

Stomach
gastrin
bombesin
vaso-active intestinal peptide (VIP)
somatostatin
substance P

Pancreatic Islet
insulin
glucagon
somatostatin
pancreatic peptide

Duodenum and Jejunum
gastrin
VIP
secretin
cholecystokinin
somatostatin
motilin
substance P
bombesin

Ileum and Colon
VIP
glucagon-like peptides
neurotensin

CAUSES OF HYPERGASTRINAEMIA

1. Gastrinoma
2. Antral G-cell hyperplasia
3. Renal failure
4. Achlorhydria
5. Retained and isolated antrum
6. Vagotomy
7. Short bowel syndrome
8. Cimetidine administration

GUT ENDOCRINE TUMOURS THAT PRESENT WITH DIARRHOEA

1. *VIP-oma (Werner Morrison syndrome, with hypokalaemia and achlorhydria)
2. Gastrinoma (Zollinger-Ellison syndrome, with intractable peptic ulcers and high gastric acid)
3. Carcinoid tumour (with flush, heart lesions and asthma)
4. Glucagonoma (with necrolytic migratory erythema, diabetes and stomatitis)
5. Somatostatinoma (with flush, diabetes and hypochlorhydria)

*VIP = vasoactive intestinal peptide

FURTHER READING

Bloom S 1979 Medicine, 3rd series, 15: 733
Buchanan K D 1980 British Journal of Hospital Medicine 24: 190
Thomas W E G 1981 Hospital Update 7: 753

Haematology

NORMAL VALUES IN HAEMATOLOGY

See note on SI units on page 194
Imperial units are given in parentheses

Haemoglobin
Men   13.0–18.0 g/dl (g. %)
Women   11.5–16.5 g/dl (g. %)

Red cells
Men $4.5-6.5 \times 10^{12}$/l (4.5–6.5 million/c.mm)
Women $3.9-5.6 \times 10^{12}$/l (3.9–5.6 million/c.mm)

Haematocrit (PCV)
Men   0.40–0.54
Women   0.36–0.47

Mean cell volume (MCV)
Adults 76–96 fl(cμ)

Mean cell haemoglobin (MCH)
Adults 27–32 pg

Mean corpuscular haemoglobin concentration (MCHC)
Adults 31–35 g/dl (g. %)

Leucocytes
Adults $4-10 \times 10^{9}$/l. (4000–10 000/c.mm)
Differential: Neutrophils 2500–7500 $\times 10^{6}$/l
              Lymphocytes 1500–3500 $\times 10^{6}$/l
              Monocytes 200–800 $\times 10^{6}$/l
              Eosinophils 40–440 $\times 10^{6}$/l
              Basophils 0–100 $\times 10^{6}$/l

Platelets
$150-400 \times 10^{9}$/l (150 000–400 000/c.mm)

Plasma viscosity
1.50–1.72 cp.

Parallels E.S.R. but is unaffected by age, sex or anaemia

E.S.R. (Westergren)
Men—up to 5 mm/h
Women—up to 7 mm/h

FURTHER READING

Cawley J C, McNicol G P 1979 British Journal of Hospital Medicine 22: 158

RED CELL SHAPE

Cell types	Causes
1. Echinocyte ('Burr' cell)	1. Uraemia
	2. Ca stomach or bleeding peptic ulcer
	3. Post transfusion with old blood
	4. Low-potassium red cells
	5. Pyruvate kinase deficiency
2. Stomatocyte ('Mouth' cell)	1. Hereditary stomatocytosis
	2. Liver disease
	3. RBC sodium-pump defect
3. Codocyte ('Target' cell)	1. Obstructive liver disease
'Target' on dried film	2. Haemoglobinopathies
	3. Thalassaemia
	4. Iron deficiency
Bell shaped on scanning electron microscopy	5. Post-splenectomy
	6. L.C.A.T. deficiency
4. Acanthocyte ('Spur' cell)	1. Abetalipoproteinaemia
	2. Alcoholic liver disease
	3. Post-splenectomy
	4. Malabsorption
5. Spherocyte ('Spherical' cell)	1. Hereditary spherocytosis
	2. Immune haemolytic anaemia
	3. Heinz body haemolytic anaemia
	4. Post-transfusion
	5. Water-dilution anaemia
	6. Fragmentation haemolysis

Cell Types	Causes
6. Elliptocyte ('Oval' cell)	1. Hereditary elliptocytosis 2. Thalassaemia 3. Iron deficiency 4. Myelophthistic anaemia 5. Megaloblastic anaemia
7. Schizocyte ('Helmet' cell)	1. Microangiopathic haemolytic anaemia 2. Heart valve haemolysis (e.g. prosthesis) 3. Severe burns or calcification 4. March haemoglobinuria
8. Drepanocyte ('Sickle' cell) Varying spiculated shapes e.g. 'Sickle' or 'Holly-leaf'	Haemoglobinopathies, SS, S-trait, SC, etc.
9. Dacryocyte ('Teardrop' cell)	1. Myelofibrosis with myeloid metaplasia 2. Myelophthistic anaemia 3. Thalassaemia
10. Leptocyte ('Wafer' cell)	1. Thalassaemia 2. Obstructive liver disease

N.B. Myelophthistic anaemia is due to a disrupted vascular pattern of the marrow. Causes include metastasis, lymphoma, myelofibrosis and T.B.

FURTHER READING

Lessin L S, Klug P P, Jensen W N 1976 Advances in Internal Medicine 21: 451

RBC abnormalities produced by absent spleen
1. Target cells
2. Acanthocytes
3. Schizocytes
4. Howell-Jolly bodies

RED CELL INCLUSION BODIES

Howell-Jolly bodies
Nuclear remnants seen as small dense purple particles at the periphery.

Causes
1. Splenectomy and splenic atrophy (p. 92)
2. Dyshaemopoietic states: leukaemia, megoblastic anaemia, etc.

Pappenheimer bodies
Fe-containing granules in siderocytes

Causes
1. Sideroblastic anaemia (q.v.)
2. Haemolytic anaemia, esp. after splenectomy

Heinz bodies
Occur in reticulocyte preparations as peripheral rounded dark blue bodies (globin denatured by oxidants)

Causes
1. Haemolytic anaemia due to oxidant drugs and chemicals
2. RBC enzyme defects, e.g. G6PD deficiency
3. Rare haemoglobinopathies ('unstable haemoglobins' e.g. Hb Koln) after splenectomy

HYPOCHROMIC ANAEMIA

Causes of hypochromic anaemia other than Fe deficiency
1. Infection
2. Rh. arthritis
3. Uraemia
5. Malignancy
} though more often normochromic
5. Thalassaemia major and minor
6. Sideroblastic anaemia (q.v.)

Causes of sideroblastic anaemia
(Defined as hypochromic anaemia with 'ring sideroblasts' in the marrow)
1. *Hereditary*
   Usually sex-linked. May or may not respond to pyridoxine
2. *Idiopathic*
3. *Drugs*
   (i) Alcohol
   (ii) Antituberculous drugs
   (iii) Chloramphenicol
4. *Lead poisoning*

(contd)

5. *Myeloproliferative disease*
6. *Haemolytic anaemia*
7. *Miscellaneous non-haematological disorders*
    (i) Malabsorption
    (ii) Infections
    (iii) Collagen-vascular disease
    (iv) Cutaneous porphyria

FURTHER READING

White J M 1974 In: Hardisty R M, Weatherall D J (eds) Blood and its
    disorders. Blackwell, Oxford, p 808

Haematological effects of lead poisoning
1. Anaemia
2. Basophilic stippling
3. Reticulocytosis
4. Erythroid hyperplasia and 'ring sideroblasts' in marrow
5. Increased Se Fe in adults
6. 'Fast' Hb (on electrophoresis) in children with Fe deficiency

FURTHER READING

White J M 1974 In: Hardisty R M, Weatherall D J (eds) Blood and its
    disorders. Blackwell, Oxford, p 821

HAEMOLYTIC ANAEMIA

CAUSES

1. **Congenital RBC defect**
    (i) Hereditary spherocytosis, elliptocytosis, stomatocytosis
    (ii) Hereditary non-spherocytic haemolytic anaemia
        Enzyme deficiency
        Thalassaemia (p. 81)
        Haemoglobinopathy, e.g. sickle-cell
        Idiopathic
    (iii) Acanthocytosis with abeta-lipoproteinaemia

2. **Acquired RBC defect**
    (i) Paroxysmal nocturnal haemoglobinuria
    (ii) Burns, radiation
    (iii) Secondary to RBC metabolic defect, e.g. megaloblastic
        anaemia or iron deficiency
    (iv) Secondary to other systemic disease, e.g. liver disease or
        vitamin E deficiency
    (v) Drugs and toxins (p. 80)

3. Immune mechanisms
  (i) Transfusion reactions
  (ii) Haemolytic disease of newborn
  (iii) Cold agglutinins (IgM, e.g. mycoplasmal pneumonia)
  (iv) Cold haemolysins (IgG, e.g. syphilis)
  (v) Autoantibodies (IgG)
      Idiopathic
      Leukaemia, lymphoma or carcinoma ⎫ 'warm' antibodies
      SLE or rheumatoid disease   ⎭
  (vi) Drugs (p. 80)

4. Infections
  (i) Septicaemia
  (ii) Malaria (especially Blackwater fever)
  (iii) Bartonellosis (Oroya fever)
  (iv) Clostridium welchii

5. Mechanical trauma
  (i) Cardiac—openheart surgery, prosthetic valve, etc.
  (ii) Microangiopathic haemolytic anaemia (q.v.)
  (iii) March haemoglobinuria

6. Hypersplenism

FURTHER READING

Flaherty T, Geary C G 1979 British Journal of Hospital Medicine 22: 334
Wiley J S 1979 Medicine, 3rd series, 28: 1468

CAUSES OF MICROANGIOPATHIC HAEMOLYTIC ANAEMIA (MHA)

  1. 'Haemolytic uraemic syndrome' Thrombocytopenia, acute
     renal failure and MHA (usually in infants)
  2. Thrombotic thrombocytopenic purpura (Moschowitz)
  3. Renal cortical necrosis
  4. Acute glomerulonephritis
  5. Eclampsia, or post-partum
  6. Malignant hypertension
  7. Disseminated carcinomatosis
  8. SLE or polyarteritis
In some cases the haemolysis is due to disseminated intravascular
coagulation

FURTHER READING

Gordon-Smith E C 1974 In: Hardisty R M, Weatherall D J (eds) Blood and its
    disorders. Blackwell, Oxford, p 763

HAEMOLYTIC ANAEMIA DUE TO DRUGS AND CHEMICALS

1. Chemicals with direct toxicity
- (i) Arsine, lead, chlorate, naphthalene
- (ii) Venoms, e.g. snake, spider
- (iii) Plant toxins, e.g. male fern

2. Drugs with direct toxicity
- Phenacetin abuse

3. Drugs with an immunological effect
- (i) Auto-immune (Antibodies directed against intrinsic R.B.C. antigens)
  - Methyl-dopa
  - Mefenamic acid
- (ii) Immune (Antibodies directed against the drug)
  - Penicillin in large doses
  - Cephalothin
  - Quinidine

4. Drugs acting on defective RBCs
- (i) Hereditary enzymopathies (e.g. deficiency of G6PD, glutathione reductase, glutathione synthetase, etc.)
  - Antimalarials, especially primaquine
  - Sulphonamides
  - Sulphones, especially dapsone
  - Antipyretics
  - Analgesics
  - Nitrofurans
  - Favism (broad beans)
- (ii) Unstable haemoglobinopathies (e.g. Hb Koln, Hb Zurich)

FURTHER READING

De Gruchy G C 1975 Drug-induced blood disorders. Blackwell, Oxford, p 156
Pettit J, Hoffbrand V 1975 Medicine, 2nd series, 6: 269

Clinical manifestations of G6P Dehydrogenase deficiency
1. Drug-induced haemolysis
2. Infection-induced haemolysis
3. Broad bean-induced haemolysis (Favism)
4. Chronic non-spherocytic haemolysis
5. Neonatal jaundice (especially after Vit. K)

THALASSAEMIA SYNDROMES
A heterogeneous group of hereditary disorders characterised by decreased synthesis of either the α or the β chain of adult HbA ($\alpha2\beta2$).

Factors in the production of the anaemia
1. The Hb deficit produces a hypochromic microcytic anaemia
2. The relative excess of α or β chains precipitates in the red cell, forming inclusion bodies (Heinz bodies) which damage the RBC membrane and cause haemolysis
3. Folic acid deficiency
4. Mitochondrial iron deposition
5. Hypersplenism

FURTHER READING

Forget B G, Nathan D C 1976 Advances in Internal Medicine 21: 97
Weatherall D J, Clegg J B 1981 The thalassaemia syndromes. Blackwell, Oxford

CAUSES OF MEGALOBLASTIC ANAEMIA

A. Folate deficiency
1. *Inadequate diet* (esp. alcoholics and old people)
2. *Malabsorption from upper intestine* (p. 50)
3. *Increased demand*
    - (i) Infancy or pregnancy
    - (ii) Increased cell turnover
        Myeloproliferative disease
        Malignancy or lymphoma
        Chronic haemolysis
        Chronic inflammation e.g. rheumatoid disease
4. *Anti-folate drugs*
    - (i) Dihydrofolate reductase inhibitors
        Methotrexate, pyrimethamine, trimethorprim
    - (ii) Impaired absorption
        Cholestyramine, sulphasalazine
    - (iii) Uncertain mechanism
        Anticonvulsants, ethanol, oral contraceptives

B. Vitamin B$_{12}$ deficiency
1. *Malabsorption*
    - (i) Lack of intrinsic factor
        Addisonian P.A.
        Partial or total gastrectomy
        Gastric atrophy due to gastritis
        Congenital P.A. with normal mucosa
        Rarely associated with polyendocrinopathy

(contd)

(ii) General malabsorption (p. 50)
(iii) Specific B_{12} malabsorption
Ileal resection
Ileal TB, Crohn's or ulcerative colitis
Chelating agents (ingested phytates)
Rarely congenital, with proteinuria
(iv) B_{12} utilisation by bacteria or parasites
Blind-loop syndrome, diverticulosis, etc.
Diphyllobothrium latum (fish tape-worm)
2. *Inadequate diet*
Rare except in vegans and starvation
3. *Drugs*
PAS, colchicine, neomycin, metformin

C. With normal folate and B_{12}

(i)   Cytotoxic drugs e.g. hydroxyurea, cytosine arabinoside
(ii) Hereditary orotic aciduria (responds to uridine)
(iii) Erythroleukaemia

FURTHER READING

Hoffbrand V 1979 Medicine, 3rd series, 28: 1438

Causes of macrocytic anaemia with normoblastic marrow
1. Haemolysis ⎫
2. Haemorrhage ⎬ since reticulocytes are macrocytes
3. Leukaemia
4. Aplastic anaemia
5. Marrow infiltration or replacement (p. 83)
6. Sideroblastic anaemia
7. Alcohol ingestion
8. Cirrhosis
9. Myxoedema or hypopituitarism
10. Protein deficiency
11. Scurvy

Causes of reduction in normal marrow activity
1. *Nutritional defect*
(i) Fe, B_{12}, folate or pyridoxine deficiency
(ii) Kwashiorkor
2. *Endocrine defect*
(i)   Erythropoietin deficiency (renal disease)
(ii) Hypothyroidism
(iii) Hypopituitarism
3. *Haemopoietic cell defect*
(i) Aplastic anaemia (p. 84)
(ii) Red-cell aplasia

4. *Marrow infiltration*
    (i) Myelofibrosis (and osteosclerosis)
    (ii) Malignant lymphoma
    (iii) Myelomatosis
    (iv) Metastatic carcinoma
    (v) Leukaemia
    (vi) Histiocytosis X
    (vii) Lipidoses (Gaucher's, Niemann-Pick's)
    (viii) Miliary TB

FURTHER READING

Lewis S M 1974 In: Hardisty R M, Weatherall D J (eds) Blood and its disorders. Blackwell, Oxford, p 1113

LEUCOPENIA

CAUSES OF NEUTROPENIA ($< 2.5 \times 10^9$ neutrophils/l)

1. Pancytopenia (q.v.)
2. Infections
    (i) Viral
    (ii) Bacterial: typhoid, brucellosis, miliary TB, overwhelming septicaemia
    (iii) Rickettsial: typhus
    (iv) Protozoal: malaria, kala-azar
3. Drugs causing selective neutropenia: thiouracil, etc.
4. Megaloblastic anaemia
5. Hypothyroidism, thyrotoxicosis, hypopituitarism
6. Cirrhosis
7. Alcoholism
8. Idiopathic (chronic or periodic)

CAUSES OF PANCYTOPENIA

1. Aplastic anaemia (p. 84)
2. Acute leukaemia (in subleukaemic phase)
3. Marrow infiltration:
    (i) Malignant lymphoma
    (ii) Metastatic carcinoma
    (iii) Myelomatosis
    (iv) Myelosclerosis (in late stages)
4. Hypersplenism
5. Pernicious anaemia
6. SLE
7. Rarely disseminated TB

Types of aplastic anaemia
A. *With thrombocytopenia* (WCC may be low or normal)
  1. Chronic acquired
    (i) Idiopathic
    (ii) Drugs or toxins
      Dose-related e.g. benzene, cytotoxics
      Idiosyncratic e.g. chloramphenicol, phenylbutazone
    (iii) Irradiation
  2. Transient, following infection (especially hepatitis)
  3. Congenital pancytopenia (Fanconi's)

N.B. (a) Pancytopenic aplastic anaemia may be complicated by paroxysmal nocturnal haemoglobinuria or leukaemia.
    (b) Chloramphenicol may produce either an early dose-related reversible marrow depression or, more rarely, an idiosyncratic severe aplastic anaemia of late onset.

B. *Red cell aplasia* (with normal WCC and platelets)
  1. Chronic acquired
    (i) Idiopathic
    (ii) Immune, with thymoma and myasthenia gravis
  2. Secondary to renal disease
  3. Associated with haemolysis, infection or riboflavin deficiency
  4. Congenital (Diamond-Blackfan)

FURTHER READING

Camitta B M et al 1982 New England Journal of Medicine 306: 645
Geary C G 1979 British Journal of Hospital Medicine 21: 392
Gordon-Smith E 1979 Medicine, 3rd series, 28: 1454

LEUCOCYTOSIS

Causes of leucocytosis ($> 10 \times 10^9$/l in adults)
  1. Physiological
    (ii) Infancy
    (ii) Pregnancy and post-partum
  2. Infection
  3. Haemorrhage
  4. Trauma, burns, surgery
  5. Myeloproliferative disease
  6. Malignancy
  7. Myocardial infarction and paroxysmal tachycardia
  8. Drugs: steroids, digitalis, adrenaline
  9. Chemicals: lead, mercury, carbon monoxide
 10. 'Collagen vascular' disease

11. Metabolic disturbances: renal failure, gout, diabetic coma, eclampsia, etc.
12. Miscellaneous: haemolysis, Se. sickness, acute anoxia, spider venom, etc.

Causes of myeloid leukaemoid reaction (WCC $> 50 \times 10^9$/l or myelocytes or myeloblasts present in peripheral blood)
1. Infections, esp. in children and after splenectomy
2. Leuco-erythroblastic anaemia (q.v.)
3. Malignancy
4. Acute haemolysis

Causes of leuco-erythroblastic anaemia
1. Metastases to bone
2. Myelosclerosis
3. Myelomatosis
4. Malignant lymphoma
5. Marble bone disease (Albers-Schonberg)
6. Gaucher's, Niemann-Pick's, Histiocytosis X

Causes of lymphocytosis ($> 3.5 \times 10^9$/l)
1. Infections
    (i) Viral: infectious mononucleosis; infective hepatitis; infectious lymphocytosis, influenza, exanthemata
    (ii) Bacterial: pyogenic infections in young children, convalescence from acute infections, pertussis, typhoid, brucellosis, TB, Sy.
    (iii) Protozoal: toxoplasmosis
2. Lymphatic leukaemia
3. Miscellaneous
    (i) Myasthenia gravis
    (ii) Thyrotoxicosis
    (iii) Hypopituitarism
    (iv) Carcinoma
    (v) Myelomatosis
4. Physiological in early childhood

Causes of eosinophilia ($> 440 \times 10^6$/l)
1. Allergy to food or drugs
2. Parasites: Hookworm, tapeworm, hydatid, ascaris, bilharzia, strongyloides, filaria, trichina, etc.
3. Skin disease
    (i) Scabies
    (ii) Dermatitis herpetiformis
    (iii) Atopic eczema
    (iv) Erythema neonatorum
4. Bronchopulmonary eosinophilia (p. 34)

(contd)

5. Post-infectious rebound
6. Blood dyscrasias, including eosinophilic leukaemia
7. Malignancy, especially Hodgkin's
8. Eosinophilic granuloma
9. Post-splenectomy
10. Rheumatoid disease with extra-articular involvement

Causes of monocytosis ($> 800 \times 10^6/l$)
   Infectious
   Viral—Infectious mononucleosis
   Rickettsial—Rocky Mountain spotted fever
   Bacterial—Listeria monocytogenes, TB, brucellosis, typhoid
   Protozoal—Malaria, kala-azar, trypanosomiasis
2. Hodgkin's disease
3. Monocytic leukaemia

HODGKIN'S DISEASE

The Rye classification
1. Lymphocytic predominance (Best prognosis)
2. Nodular sclerosis
3. Mixed cellularity
4. Lymphocytic depletion (Worst prognosis)

Essential criteria for the histological diagnosis of Hodgkin's disease
1. Complete or partial destruction of the nodal architecture (reticulin stain)
2. Presence of abnormal reticulum cells
3. Presence of Sternberg-Reed giant cells

Clinical staging

Stage	Description
I	Disease limited to one anatomical region
II	(1) Disease limited to two contiguous anatomical regions on same side of the diaphragm
	(2) Disease in more than two anatomical regions or in two non-contiguous regions on same side of diaphragm
III	Disease on both sides of diaphragm but limited to involvement of lymph nodes, spleen and Waldeyer's ring
IV	Involvement of any tissue or organ other than lymph nodes, spleen or Waldeyer's ring

All stages are subclassified as A or B to indicate the absence or presence, respectively, of symptoms

FURTHER READING

Cooper I 1979 Medicine, 3rd series, 29: 1493
Harrison C V 1975 In: Harrison C V, Weinbren K (eds) Recent advances in
    pathology—9, Churchill Livingstone, Edinburgh, p 73

NON-HODGKIN'S LYMPHOMATA

Identification of more cell types in the lymph nodes has led to increasingly complex classifications, but their relationship to prognosis remains uncertain. The following classification incorporates some of the newer concepts but avoids much of the controversial terminology.

	Traditional name
A. *Follicular lymphoma*	
1. Cells predominantly small	
2. Mixed small and large cells	Follicular lymphoma
3. Cells predominantly large	
B. *Diffuse lymphoma*	
1. Lymphocytic (i) Well-differentiated	
(ii) Intermediate	Lympho-sarcoma
(iii) Poorly differentiated	
(iv) Mixed small and large cells	
2. 'Undifferentiated' large cell	Reticulum cell sarcoma
3. Histiocytic (shown by E. M. and histochemistry)	
4. Plasma cell	Plasmacytoma
C. Primary cutaneous T cell lymphoma	Mycosis fungoides
D. Unclassified	

FURTHER READING

Copper I 1979 Medicine, 3rd series, 29: 1493
Crowther D, Scarffe J H 1977 In: Baron D N, Compston N, Dawson A M
    (eds) Recent advances in medicine—17. Churchill Livingstone, Edinburgh,
    p 41
Nathwani B 1979 Cancer 44: 347

CLASSIFICATION OF LEUKAEMIA

ACUTE ('*Poorly differentiated*')

1. Acute myeloid (AML)
Subdivided according to predominant cells
  (i) Myeloblastic
  (ii) Promyelocytic
  (iii) Myelocytic
  (iv) Myelomonocytic
  (v) Monocytic
  (vi) Erythro-leukaemic

2. Acute lymphoblastic (ALL)
  (i) Null cell (80%)
  (ii) T cell
  (iii) B cell
Distinguished from other types by
  (i) peak incidence at 3–5 yr
  (ii) better response to treatment, with long remission
  (iii) mature cells with normal morphology

CHRONIC ('*Well-differentiated*')

1. Myeloid
  (i) Chronic granulocytic (CGL)
      Most are Philadelphia chromosome positive. In the atypical
      juvenile form, Hb F is increased
  (ii) Chronic myelomonocytic (with high neutrophil count)
  (iii) Chronic monocytic (with normal or low neutrophil count)
  (iv) Neutrophilic (very rare)

2. Lymphocytic
  (i) Chronic lymphocytic (CLL)
  (ii) Chronic leukaemia with lymphoma
      e.g. Waldenstrom's macroglobulinaemia
          Follicular lymphoma
          Diffuse lymphocytic lymphoma
          Sézary syndrome (with pruritus, erythroderma and
          circulating Sézary T cells)

FURTHER READING

Cawley J J, Goldstone A H 1975 Hospital Update 1: 719
Chessells Judith M, Powles R 1979 Medicine, 3rd series, 29: 1477
Goldman J M 1979 Medicine, 3rd series 29: 1486

MYELOPROLIFERATIVE DISEASES

1. Primary polycythaemia vera
2. Myelofibrosis
3. Thrombocythaemia
4. Erythroleukaemia (Di Guglielmo)
5. Atypical myeloproliferative disorders
   Some authorities now exclude leukaemia from the
   myeloproliferative disorders, although transitions can occur as
   follows:

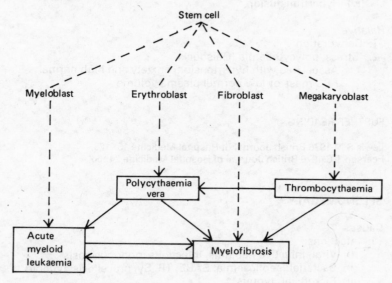

FURTHER READING

Whitehouse J M 1975 Medicine, 2nd eries, 30: 1687

CAUSES OF POLYCYTHAEMIA

Absolute
1. Idiopathic PC Vera
2. Secondary
   (i) Hypoxic
       High altitude
       Cardiac or pulmonary disease
       Cerebral (decreased respiratory drive)
       Obesity (Pickwickian syndrome)
       Methaemoglobinaemia and sulphaemoglobinaemia

(*contd*)

    (ii) Erythropoietin
            Kidney disease (p. 158)
            Carcinoma of liver
            Cerebellar haemangioblastoma
            Uterine myomata
            Virilizing syndromes
            Phaeochromocytoma
   (iii) Benign familial, due to abnormal Hb with either high
            oxygen affinity or excess methaemoglobin
   (iv) Hypertransfusion

Relative
1. Dehydration
2. 'Stress' polycythaemia (Gaisböck)
            Associated with hypertension, anxiety and high normal
            RBC mass or low normal plasma volume

FURTHER READING

Lewis S M 1976 British Journal of Hospital Medicine 15: 125
Pearson T C 1979 British Journal of Hospital Medicine 24: 66

SPLENOMEGALY

Causes
1. Infections
        (i) Viral- infective hepatitis, infectious mononucleosis
       (ii) Bacterial: septicaemia, SABE, TB, Sy, brucellosis, typhoid
      (iii) Rickettsial: typhus
      (iv) Fungal: histoplasmosis
       (v) Protozoal: malaria, kala-azar, trypanosomiasis
      (vi) Parasitic: hydatid
2. Blood dyscrasia
        (i) Leukaemia
       (ii) Haemolytic anaemia
      (iii) Myelofibrosis
      (iv) Polycythaemia vera
       (v) Occasionally in ITP, myelomatosis, megaloblastic anaemia
            and chronic Fe-deficiency anaemia
3. Malignant lymphomas
4. Miscellaneous
        (i) Portal hypertension
       (ii) Lipoid storage disease
      (iii) Benign tumours and cysts
      (iv) Occasionally in SLE, sarcoidosis, amyloidosis, Rh. arthritis,
            hyperthyroidism, etc.

Causes of a huge spleen

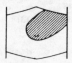

Chronic myeloid leukaemia
Myelofibrosis
Malaria
Kala-azar
Gaucher's disease
Lymphocytic lymphoma

Look for evidence of iliac bone biopsy as this suggests myelofibrosis

Causes of moderately large spleen

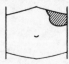

Above 6
+Storage diseases
    Haemolytic anaemias
    Portal hypertension
    Leukaemias

Causes of a just palpable spleen

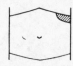

Above 10
+all other causes of
splenomegaly (q.v.)

FURTHER READING

Billinghurst J R 1978 British Journal of Hospital Medicine 20: 413

HYPERSPLENISM

(reduction of 1 or more of the formed elements of the blood due to functional hyperactivity of the spleen)

Causes

1. Portal hypertension
2. Malignant lymphoma
3. Chronic lymphatic leukaemia or myelofibrosis, especially after repeated transfusions
4. Lipidoses (Gaucher's, Niemann-Pick's)
5. Sarcoidosis
6. Chronic infection
    T.B., brucellosis, bacterial endocarditis
    Kala-azar and malaria
7. Rheumatoid disease (especially Felty's syndrome)

8. Red cell disorders
     Congenital e.g. thalassaemia, spherocytosis
     Acquired e.g. auto-immune haemolysis, paroxysmal
     nocturnal haemoglobinuria
9. Idiopathic

FURTHER READING

Richards J D M 1976 British Journal of Hospital Medicine 15: 505
Richmond J 1980 British Journal of Hospital Medicine 24: 405

Common indications for splenectomy
1. Surgical, including trauma
2. Hereditary spherocytosis
3. Chronic ITP
4. Hypersplenism causing symptoms

Other indications
5. Acquired haemolytic anaemia
6. Acute ITP
7. Hereditary elliptocytosis
8. Myelofibrosis
9. Chronic lymphatic leukaemia
10. Malignant lymphomas
11. Thalassaemia major

ABSENCE OR ATROPHY OF SPLEEN

Causes
1. Splenectomy
2. Splenic infarct (including sickle cell disease)
3. Coeliac syndrome (including dermatitis herpetiformis)
4. Tropical sprue
5. Ulcerative colitis
6. Fanconi's anaemia
7. Congenital absence

PLATELETS

Causes of thrombocytopenia ($< 150 \times 10^9$/l)
1. *Decreased production*
     (i) Marrow aplasia e.g. drugs or toxins
     (ii) Marrow infiltration e.g. leukaemia
     (iii) Uraemia
     (iv) Megaloblastic anaemia
     (v) Alcoholism

2. *Decreased survival*
   Immunological
   (i) Idiopathic thrombocytopenic purpura (ITP)
   (ii) Drugs affecting platelets selectively e.g. quinine, sulphona-
        mides, thiazides, rifampicin, indomethacin, phenylbuta-
        zone
   (iii) Blood transfusion with incompatible platelets
   (iv) 'Secondary' thrombocytopenia—
        a. SLE
        b. Chronic lymphatic leukaemia
        c. Auto-immune haemolytic anaemia with ITP (Evans' syn-
           drome)
   Increased consumption
   (i) Disseminated intra-vascular coagulation (p. 100)
   (ii) Thrombotic thrombocytopenic purpura (Moschcowitz's)
   (iii) Large haemangiomata
   (iv) Infections—R.M. Spotted Fever
                   Typhus
                   Bacterial endocarditis
                   Meningococcal septicaemia
                   Exanthemata
3. *Sequestration*—Hypersplenism, hypothermia
4. *Dilution*—Massive transfusion of stored blood
5. *Loss*—Massive haemorrhage

In some conditions, e.g. uraemia there may be several mechanisms
In neonates and children the following must also be considered:
1. Rare congenital disorders
   (i) Fanconi's aplastic anaemia (with multiple congenital ano-
        malies)
   (ii) Familial thrombocytopenia
   (iii) Megakaryocyte aplasia
   (iv) Aldrich-Wiskott syndrome (with eczema and immunologic-
        al deficiencies)
   (v) May Hegglin anomaly (with giant platelets)
2. Mothers with ITP, SLE or drug purpura
3. Viral or parasitic: Congenital rubella syndrome
                      Toxoplasmosis
                      Cytomegalic inclusion disease
4. Cyanotic congenital heart disease
5. Haemolytic uraemia syndrome

FURTHER READING

Sanderson J H, Goldstone A H 1977 Hospital Update 3: 249

Causes of qualitative platelet defects (i.e. platelet dysfunction)

A. *Congenital*
  1. Hereditary thrombasthenia (Glanzmann)
     Impaired platelet aggregation
  2. Congenital abnormalities of platelet release or adhesion
  3. Giant platelet syndrome (Bernard-Soulier)
  4. Associated with other hereditary disease
     (i) von Willebrand's disease, and some haemophilia
     (ii) Hermansky-Pudlak (with albinism)
     (iii) Cutis hyperelastica (Ehlers-Danlos)
     (iv) Wiskott-Aldrich

B. *Acquired*
  1. Drugs
     (i) Aspirin
     (ii) Indomethacin
     (iii) Phenylbutazone
     (iv) Streptokinase
     (v) High M.W. dextran infusion
  2. Systemic diseases
     (i) Uraemia
     (ii) Liver disease
     (iii) Dysproteinaemia
     (iv) Scurvy
     (v) SLE
  3. Myeloproliferative disease, esp. thrombocythaemia (excessive platelets of abnormal morphology)
  4. Aplastic anaemia or leukaemia

FURTHER READING

Bowie E J W, Owen C A 1977 In: Poller L (ed) Recent advances in blood coagulation—2. Churchill Livingstone, Edinburgh, p 59
Hellem A J 1976 Advances in Internal Medicine 17: 171

Tests of platelet dysfunction in thrombasthenia and von Willebrand's disease

	Thrombasthenia	von Willebrand's disease
Platelet aggregation		
1. To ADP	Absent	Normal
2. To collagen	Absent	Normal
3. To ristocetin	Absent	Absent
Platelet adhesion to glass beads	Low	Low or normal

FURTHER READING

Brozovic M, Machin S 1977 Hospital Update 3: 203

Causes of thrombocytosis (Increased platelets, $> 400 \times 10^9/l$)
1. Haemorrhage, surgery, trauma
2. Splenectomy or splenic atrophy
3. Myeloproliferative disorders, especially megakaryocytic leukaemia and haemorrhagic thrombocythaemia
4. Chronic inflammatory disease
5. Malignancy
6. 'Rebound' after recovery from haemolysis or treatment of pernicious anaemia
7. Chronic renal disease

FURTHER READING

Sanderson J H, Goldstone A H 1977 Hospital Update 3: 249

Conditions predisposing to thrombosis

A. *Localised*
1. Stasis (tight bandages, etc.)
2. Damaged vessel wall
   (i) Infection
   (ii) Atheroma
   (iii) Trauma

B. *Generalised*
1. Thrombocytosis
2. Prolonged bed rest
3. Pregnancy and puerperium
4. Oral contraceptives
5. Hyperviscosity of blood (dysproteinaemia or polycythaemia)
6. Smoking
7. Congestive heart failure
8. Chronic infection
9. Blood group A1
10. Family history of thrombosis

FURTHER READING

O'Brien J R 1977 In: Poller L (ed) Recent advances in blood coagulation—2. Churchill Livingstone, Edinburgh, p 241

VESSEL DEFECTS

Causes of bleeding due to defects of vessels or supportive tissues

A. *Acquired*
  1. *Vasculitis* (p. 178), especially Henoch-Schönlein purpura and allergic vasculitis due to drugs
  2. *Defect in connective tissue*
     (i) Senile purpura
     (ii) Cushing's disease or glucocorticoid therapy
     (iii) Scurvy (controversial, since platelets are defective)
  3. *Amyloidosis* (primary and secondary)
  4. *Anoxia*
     (i) Dysproteinaemia
     (ii) Fat embolism
  5. *Infections*
     (i) Bacterial endocarditis
     (ii) Septicaemia
     (iii) Viral and rickettsial infections
  6. *Dermatoses*
     (i) Eczema
     (ii) Pigmented purpuric dermatosis (Schamberg, etc.)
     (iii) Drug-induced capillaropathy, especially carbromal
     (iv) Simple easy bruising
     (v) Erythrocyte auto-sensitisation ('psychogenic' purpura)

B. *Congenital*
  1. Hereditary haemorrhagic telangiectasia
  2. Hereditary capillary fragility
  3. Pseudo-xanthoma elasticum
  4. Cutis hyperelastica (Ehlers-Danlos)

COAGULATION

The coagulation cascade
Several new factors (Fletcher, Fitzgerald, Passovoy) involved in the initial phase of intrinsic coagulation have been described, but their role is not fully understood.

Factor XII is also involved in:
  1. activation of fibrinolysis
  2. conversion of kallikreinogen to kallikrein
  3. formation of plasma permeability factor

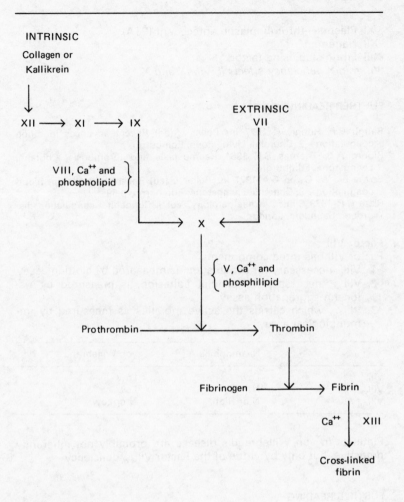

Blood coagulation factors
   I   Fibrinogen
   II   Prothrombin
   III   (Platelet lipid)
   IV   (Ca^{++})
   V   Proaccelerin (labile)
   VI   —
   VII   Proconvertin (stable)
   VIII   Anti-haemophilic globulin
   IX   Christmas factor
   X   Stuart-Prower

(contd)

XI   Plasma—thromboplastin antecedent (PTA)
XII Hageman
XIII Fibrin-stabilising factor
Vitamin K deficiency affects II, VII, IX and X

FURTHER READING

Baugh R F, Hougie C 1977 In: Poller L (ed) Recent advances in blood coagulation—2. Churchill Livingstone, Edinburgh, p 1
Bloom A L, Thomas D P 1981 Haemostasis and thrombosis. Churchill Livingstone, Edinburgh
Bowie E J W, Owen C A 1977 In: Poller L (ed) Recent advances in blood coagulation—2. Churchill Livingstone, Edinburgh, p 59
Rizza C R 1979 Clinics in haematology, Vol 9. Congenital coagulation disorders. Saunders, London

Factor VIII
Factor VIII has three components
  1. VIII_c, necesssary for coagulation, is measured by clotting assay
  2. VIII_{vw}, necessary for platelet adhesion, is measured by ristocetin aggregation assay
  3. VIII_{Ag}, which carries the active moieties, is measured by immunological assay

	Haemophilia A	von Willebrand's
VIII_c	Low	Low
VIII_{vw}	N	Low
VIII_{Ag}	N or High	N or Low

Platelets in von Willebrand's disease are probably not inherently defective, but only by virtue of the Factor VIII_{vw} deficiency

FURTHER READING

Brozovic M, Machin S 1977 Hospital Update 3: 203
Rickard K A, York J R, MacDonald D 1979 Medicine, 3rd series, 28: 1421
Sanderson J H, Goldstone A H 1977 Hospital Update 3: 249

SCREENING TESTS FOR A BLEEDING DISORDER

1. **Blood count and film**
   To detect leukaemia and assess platelet number, size and shape

2. **Platelet count**

3. **Bleeding time** (with Duke's method, normal < 7 min.). Useful in diagnosis of von Willebrand's disease

4. **Hess test**, with sphygmomanometer cuff at c.100 mmHg for 5 min.

5. **One-stage prothrombin time** (N. 12–15 sec.)
   Tests the extrinsic system
   Prolonged in
   (i) Deficiency of II, V, VII or X
   (ii) Severe fibrinogen deficiency
   (iii) Presence of some inhibitors e.g. heparin or fibrin degradation products

6. **Activated partial thromboplastin time (APTT)**
   Tests the intrinsic system (especially VIII and IX)
   Uses kaolin in place of 'exposed collagen'

7. **Calcium thrombin time** (N. 10–20 sec.)
   Prolonged in
   (i) Fibrinogen deficiency
   (ii) Presence of some inhibitors, e.g. heparin

8. **Prothrombin consumption index**
   Very sensitive test which detects both platelet and coagulation abnormalities

9. **Fibrin degradation products**
   Increased in fibrinolysis
   Normal screening tests do not exclude vascular defects, e.g. senile purpura or mild coagulation factor deficiency, e.g. VIII (Haemophilia A) or IX (Haemophilia B)

FURTHER READING

Brozovic M, Machin S 1977 Hospital Update 3: 203
Lewis J H, Spero J A, Hasbida U 1978 Bleeding disorders: discussions in patient management. Kimpton, London
Rizza C R 1979 Clinics in haematology, Vol. 9. Congenital coagulation disorders. Saunders, London

CAUSES OF FIBRINOGEN DEFICIENCY (< 1.5 g/l)

In many cases there are multiple causes.

Acquired
1. *Impaired formation* e.g. liver disease
2. *Increased consumption* ('disseminated intra-vascular coagulation', q.v.)
3. *Increased destruction* (excessive fibrinolysis)
   Usually secondary to 'disseminated intra-vascular coagulation'

Congenital
Very rare

DISSEMINATED INTRAVASCULAR COAGULATION

This is characterised by excessive formation of fibrinogen derivatives, usually due to increased proteolysis. There may be bleeding or thrombosis of any severity.

Causes
1. 'Shock', esp. Gram neg. septicaemia and anaphylaxis
2. Other infections, e.g. TB, viral and fungal
3. Obstetric
   Premature placental separation
   Retention of dead fetus
   Amniotic embolism
   Fetal death due to Rh incompatibility
4. Major surgery, especially with extra-corporeal shunts
5. Incompatible blood transfusion
6. Miscellaneous
   Leukaemia or carcinomatosis
   Liver, renal or prostatic disease
   Pulmonary embolism
   Snake venom

Minimum laboratory criteria for diagnosis
At least 2 of the following:
1. Increased fibrin degradation products in serum
2. Decreased plasma fibrinogen
3. Prolonged thrombin clotting time
4. Positive ethanol gelation

In severe cases there may be a decrease in platelets, and factors II, V and VIII

FURTHER READING

Cash J 1977 In: Poller L (ed) Recent advances in blood coagulation—2.
  Churchill Livingstone, Edinburgh, p 293
Chesterman C N 1979 Medicine, 3rd series, 28: 1428
Preston F E 1979 British Journal of Hospital Medicine 21: 232

CAUSES OF HYPOPROTHROMBINAEMIA

1. *Vitamin K deficiency*
   - (i) Dietary deficiency (uncommon)
   - (ii) Defective synthesis by intestinal bacteria, e.g. in neonates or after antibiotics
   - (iii) Malabsorption, e.g. biliary obstruction
   - (iv) Renal failure (probably multifactorial)
2. *Liver disease*
3. *Drugs*
   - (i) Vitamin K antagonists
   - (ii) Thiouracil, salicylates, etc.
4. *Carcinomatosis* (uncommon)
5. *Congenital* (very rare)

Conditions associated with circulating anticoagulants

1. *Anticoagulants to AHG, etc.*
   - (i) Haemophilia (? due to repeated transfusions)
   - (ii) Pregnancy, often with Rh incompatibility
   - (iii) Malignancy
   - (iv) Collagen vascular disease
   - (v) Pemphigus
   - (vi) Idiopathic
2. *Heparin-like anticoagulants*
   - (i) Irradiation
   - (ii) Cytotoxic therapy

COMPLICATIONS OF BLOOD TRANSFUSION

1. *Febrile reactions*
   - (i) Pyrogens
   - (ii) Leucocyte or platelet iso-agglutinins
   - (iii) Hypersensitivity to plasma
2. *Allergic reactions*
3. *Circulatory overload*
4. *Haemolysis.* Red cells of either donor or recipient may be affected
   - (i) Blood group incompatibility
   - (ii) Improper or overlong storage of donor blood

(*contd*)

5. *Reaction due to infected stored blood*
6. *Disease transmission*
   (i) Viral hepatitis, cytomegalovirus, Epstein Barr virus, herpes simplex
   (ii) Syphilis
   (iii) Malaria, toxoplasmosis
   (iv) Brucellosis
7. *Thrombophlebitis*
8. *Air embolism*
9. *Immunological sensitisation by compatible blood*, especially Rhesus sensitisation
10. *Transfusion siderosis*
11. *Complications of massive transfusion*
    (i) Collapse due to cold blood
    (ii) Excess citrate (exaggerates bleeding tendency)
    (iii) Excess ammonia from stored blood (exaggerates pre-coma in cirrhotics)
    (iv) Excess potassium (exaggerates hyperkalaemia in uraemic patients)
    (v) Thrombocytopenia
12. *Development of circulating anticoagulants* e.g. AHG antibody antibody

FURTHER READING

Machin S G 1979 British Journal of Hospital Medicine 21: 294
Tovey G H, Bird G W G 1974 In: Hardisty R M, Weatherall D J (eds) Blood and its disorders. Blackwell, Oxford, p 1481

Neurology

Terms which are often confused

1. *Dysphasia.* Cortical disorder in use of symbols for
   communication, whether spoken, heard, written or read
   Dysarthria. Disorder of articulation of speech
2. *Apraxia.* Inability to carry out purposive learned movements in
   absence of motor paralysis, sensory loss or ataxia
   Agnosia. Failure to recognise, whether visual, auditory or
   tactile
3. *Perseveration.* Continuation or recurrence of an activity without
   appropriate stimulus
   Verbigeration. Meaningless repetition of words or sentences
   Echolalia. Parrot-like repetition by the subject of statements or
   acts made before them
4. *Epilepsy.* A paroxysmal transitory disturbance of brain
   function, ceasing spontaneously, with a tendency to recurrence
   Myoclonus. A brief shock-like contraction of a number of
   muscle fibres, a whole muscle or several muscles, either
   simultaneously or successively
5. *Fibrillation.* Spontaneous contraction of individual muscle
   fibres (EMG finding)
   Fasciculation. Spontaneous contraction of bundles of fibres in
   the same motor unit (seen clinically)
6. *Amaurosis.* Blindness from any cause
   Amblyopia. Poor vision not due to retractive error or ocular
   disease
7. *Athetosis.* Involuntary slow coarse writhing movements,
   usually most pronounced in hand or arms
   Dystonia. Involuntary sustained twisting movements, usually
   affecting proximal muscles

BRAIN DEATH

Electroencephalography is not necessary for the diagnosis of brain death, but if an artificial life support system is to be withdrawn (e.g. for donation of organs for transplantation) the following tests should be performed by two doctors, one of whom should preferably be the Consultant in charge of the case, and the tests may need to be repeated. The interval between the tests will depend on the primary pathology and the clinical course of the disease, and it might be as long as 24 hours. The body temperature should be not less than 35 °C before the diagnostic tests are performed.

Diagnostic tests for the confirmation of brain death
All brainstem reflexes are absent:
1. Pupils fixed and do not react to light
2. No corneal reflex
3. No vestibulo-ocular reflexes (using 20 ml of ice cold water in each external auditory meatus)
4. No motor responses in the cranial nerve distribution following adequate stimulation of any somatic area
5. No gag reflex to a suction catheter passed down the trachea
6. No respiratory movements occur when the patient is disconnected from the respirator for long enough to ensure a rise in arterial pCO_2 above 50 mmHg (threshold for stimulation of respiration). Patients with pre-existing chronic respiratory insufficiency will require special consideration

FURTHER READING

Conference of Medical Royal Colleges and their Faculties in U.K. (1976)
    Lancet ii: 1069
Health Departments of Great Britain and Northern Ireland 1979 The removal
    of cadaveric organs for transplantation: a code of practice. HMSO,
    London

HARMFUL EFFECTS OF ALCOHOL (ethanol and congeners)

1. *Social complications of intoxication or alcoholism*
2. *Physical complications of acute intoxication*
    e.g. Accidents, coma, inhaled vomitus, Mallory-Weiss
        syndrome, 'hang-over'
3. *Neuro-psychiatric*
    (i) Withdrawal syndromes
        a. Tremulousness
        b. Psychoses (paranoia, hallucinations, etc.)
        c. Epilepsy (also pptd by hypoglycaemia)
        d. Delirium tremens

(ii) Nutritional deficiency syndromes
   a. Wernicke-Korsakoff syndrome
        Ophthalmoplegia with nystagmus
        Ataxia
        Confusion and dullness
        Amnesia and confabulation
   b. Peripheral neuropathy (Wallerian degeneration)
   c. Cerebellar degeneration
   d. Central pontine myelinolysis (produces bulbar palsy)
   e. Degeneration of corpus callosum
   f. Retrobulbar neuropathy ('alcoholic amblyopia')
(iii) Toxic effects
   a. Acute myositis after a drinking bout
   b. Subacute myopathy (usually proximal)
(iv) Neurological effects of liver disease
   a. Encephalopathy (p. 56)
   b. Myelopathy (esp. after porta-caval shunt)
   c. Neuropathy (mild but not rare)
(v) Psychoses
        Paranoia, hallucinations, morbid jealousy, fugue,
        increased suicide risk, etc.

4. *Gastro-intestinal*
   (i) Acute gastritis and gastric ulcer
   (ii) Fatty liver or alcoholic hepatitis
   (iii) Cirrhosis
   (iv) Pancreatitis
   (v) Malabsorption
   (vi) Increased risk of Ca. oesophagus

5. *Cardiac*
   (i) Arrhythmia
   (ii) Congestive cardiomyopathy
   (iii) Beri-beri heart disease
   (iv) Cardiomyopathy due to cobalt additives

6. *Haematological*
   Diminished haemopoiesis (RBCs, WBCs and platelets) due to
   dietary deficiency and toxic effect on marrow

7. *Metabolic*
   (i) Obesity or malnutrition
   (ii) Hypoglycaemia
   (iii) Hyperlipaemia
   (iv) Hyperuricaemia
   (v) Increased cortisol production
   (vi) Diuresis and electrolyte disturbance
   (vii) Haemochromatosis
   (viii) Porphyria cutanea tarda

8. *Increased incidence of infection*, esp. bacterial pneumonia, TB

(contd)

9. *Effects on the fetus*
    (i) Increased risk of congenital defects
        a. Microcephaly
        b. Cardiac defect
        c. Growth deficiency
        d. Mental deficiency
    (ii) Increased peri-natal mortality

FURTHER READING

Hore B D et al 1977 British Journal of Hospital Medicine 18: 106–143
Rail D L, Swash M 1982 British Journal of Hospital Medicine 8:1463

CAUSES OF DYSARTHRIA

1. *Bilateral upper motor-neurone (supranuclear) lesion of cranial nerves 9, 10 or 12 (Pseudo-bulbar palsy)*
    e.g. Cerebral ischaemia
        Motor neurone disease
        Multiple sclerosis

2. *Lower motor-neurone lesion of cranial nerves 9, 10 or 12 (Bulbar palsy)*
    e.g. Motor neurone disease
        Bulbar polio
        Medullary tumour
        Syringobulbia
        Guillain-Barré

3. *Basal ganglion lesions*
    e.g Parkinsonism
        Choreo-athetosis
        Hepato-lenticular degeneration (Wilson's)

4. *Cerebellar lesions*
    e.g Multiple sclerosis
        Toxins or drugs, especially alcohol
        Tumour

5. *Myasthenia gravis, facial muscular dystrophy and facial palsy*

6. *Oral lesions*
    e.g False teeth
        Tongue-tie
        Cleft palate

CAUSES OF EPILEPSY

1. *Idiopathic (including genetic factors)*
2. *Focal lesions*
    - (i) Birth injury
    - (ii) Tumour esp. meningioma
    - (iii) Trauma, scar
    - (iv) Vascular
        - Angiomatous malformation
        - Cerebral ischaemia or infarct
        - Acute hypertension
    - (v) Infectious
        - Encephalitis or meningitis
        - Abscess or tuberculoma
        - Neurosyphilis (p. 125)
        - Hydatid or cysticercosis
    - (vi) Primary dementias (p. 108)
    - (vii) Other neurological disease
        - Multiple sclerosis, leucodystrophies
        - Tuberose sclerosis (epiloia)
3. *Metabolic*
    - (i) Anoxia
    - (ii) Hypoglycaemia
    - (iii) Hypocalcaemia
    - (iv) Alkalosis
    - (v) Water intoxication
    - (vi) Uraemia
    - (vii) Hepatic coma
    - (viii) Lipidoses (Tay-Sachs)
    - (ix) Drugs and chemicals
        - Nikethamide, lignocaine
        - Lead poisoning
        - Cocaine
        - Ether
        - Withdrawal of alcohol or barbiturates
    - (x) Pyrexia, especially in children

CAUSES OF DISSEMINATED CNS LESIONS

1. Multiple sclerosis
2. Meningovascular syphilis
3. Multiple infarcts
4. Multiple metastases
5. Subacute combined degeneration
6. Tabes dorsalis
7. Friedreich's ataxia
8. Neuromyelitis optica
9. Diffuse sclerosis
10. Progressive multifocal leuco-encephalopathy

CAUSES OF DEMENTIA

Primary 'pre-senile' or 'senile' dementia
1. Idiopathic cerebral atrophy
2. Alzheimer's
3. Pick's
4. Creutzfeld-Jakob's transmissable dementia
5. Huntington's

Secondary
A. *Intra-cranial*
1. Tumour, especially frontal
2. Sub-dural haematoma
3. Vascular disease, esp. atheroma and multiple small infarcts due to thrombo-emboli from heart or large arteries
4. Trauma (includes repeated concussion of boxers and jockeys)
5. Infections
     (i) Encephalitis, abscess, meningitis
     (ii) Neuro-syphilis, esp. GPI
6. Multiple sclerosis and leucodystrophies
7. Neuro-lipidoses
8. Parkinsonism
9. Chronic epilepsy
10. Normal pressure hydrocephalus
11. Psychosis e.g. schizophrenia, chronic depression

B. *Extra-cranial*
1. Metabolic
     (i) Prolonged or recurrent anoxia or hypoglycaemia
     (ii) Chronic renal failure
     (iii) Hepatic failure
     (iv) Electrolyte imbalance
     (v) Carcinomatous neuropathy (p. 124)
2. Endocrine
     (i) Hypothyroidism
     (ii) Hypopituitarism
     (iii) Hypoadrenalism
     (iv) Hypo- or hyper-parathyroidism
3. Vitamin deficiency
     (i) B_{12} or folate
     (ii) Thiamine (esp. in alcoholics)
     (iii) Nicotinic acid (pellagra)
4. Drugs
     Barbiturates, cannabis, bromides, phenacetin
5. Toxins
     Alcohol, lead, manganese, arsenic, etc.

FURTHER READING

Lishman W A 1975 In: Lant A F (ed) Advanced medicine, symposium 11.
  Pitman, London, p 128

CAUSES OF COMA

1. *Head injury*
2. *Epilepsy*
3. *Drugs*
        Alcohol
        Hypnotics
        Carbon monoxide
        Aspirin
4. *Metabolic*
        Hyper- or hypo-glycaemia
        Uraemia
        Myxoedema
        Hepatic failure
        Hypoadrenalism
        Hypopituitarism
        Hypocapnia
        Electrolyte imbalance
5. *Vascular*
        Cerebral thrombosis, embolism, haemorrhage
        Hypertensive encephalopathy
        Causes of syncope (p. 18)
6. *Pressure effects*
        Space-occupying lesions
        Hydrocephalus
7. *Acute infection of CNS*
        Meningitis
        Encephalitis
        Abscess
8. *Acute systemic infection*
        Malaria
        Septicaemia
9. *Hysteria or hypnosis*
10. *Hyper- or hypothermia.*

MECHANISMS OF HEADACHE PRODUCTION

1. *Skeletal muscle contraction*, e.g. 'tension' headache
2. *Referred pain*, e.g. disease of eyes, ears, sinuses, cervical spine
3. *Arterial dilatation*
   (i) Intra-cranial, e.g. systemic infections, hypertension, nitrites, anoxia, 'hang-over', post-ictal, concussion
   (ii) Extra-cranial, e.g. migraine
4. *Traction on arteries*, e.g. raised IC pressure (haemorrhage, tumour, etc)
5. *Dilatation or traction on venous sinuses*, e.g. post-lumbar puncture
6. *Inflammation*
   (i) Intra-cranial, e.g. meningitis
   (ii) Extra-cranial, e.g. giant-cell arteritis
7. *Psychogenic*

FURTHER READING

Lance J W 1978 Mechanism and management of headache, 3rd edn. Butterworth, London

THE ANATOMY OF THE FACIAL NERVE

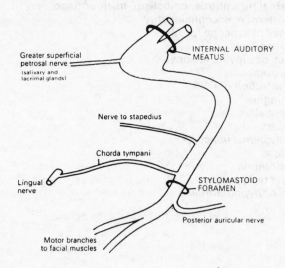

Greater superficial petrosal nerve
(salivary and lacrimal glands)

INTERNAL AUDITORY MEATUS

Nerve to stapedius

Chorda tympani

Lingual nerve

STYLOMASTOID FORAMEN

Posterior auricular nerve

Motor branches to facial muscles

Hints on localization of lesion in facial paralysis
1. Associated lesions may help
   e.g. Ipsilateral 6th nerve palsy suggests brainstem
        5th and 8th nerve lesions suggest cerebello-pontine angle
        Hyperacusis (n. to stapedius) and loss of taste (lingual n.)
        suggest bony canal
2. Paresis of frontalis muscle indicates a nuclear or infra-nuclear
   lesion
3. In supra-nuclear lesions emotional facial movements are
   occasionally retained

*N.B. Exclude myasthenia gravis and facial myopathy. They usually
produce bilateral weakness, with ptosis.*

FURTHER READING

Adour K K 1982 New England Journal of Medicine 307: 348

Causes of facial pain
1. Disease of teeth, sinuses, ear, nose or throat
2. Trigeminal neuralgia
3. Post-herpetic neuralgia
4. Migrainous neuralgia ('cluster' headache)
5. Aneurysm of post. communicating or int. carotid artery
6. Cranial arteritis
7. Raeder's paratrigeminal syndrome—Severe retro-orbital pain
   succeeded by ipsilateral miosis and ptosis
8. Superior orbital fissure syndrome—Boring retro-orbital pain
   and paresis of cranial nerves 3, 4, 5 and 6
9. Causalgia from partial 5th n. lesions
10. 'Atypical facial pain'—Constant, nagging deep pain not
    corresponding to any anatomical sensory distribution
11. Temporo-mandibular arthritis
12. Myocardial ischaemia (rarely)

FURTHER READING

Graham J G 1976 In: Peters D K (ed) Advanced medicine, symposium 12.
  Pitman, London, p 149
Zilkha K J 1979 British Journal of Hospital Medicine 21: 112

Ramsay-Hunt syndrome (geniculate herpes zoster)
1. Vesicles on auricle or anterior fauces
2. Pain in ear and mastoid region
3. Ipsilateral taste loss in anterior two-thirds tongue
4. Facial paresis or spasm
5. Deafness or dizziness
6. Hyperacusis (paralysis of n. to stapedius)

Causes of nystagmus
1. Physiological, e.g. opto-kinetic
2. Errors of refraction and macular lesions
3. Weakness of ocular muscles
4. Lesion of cranial nerves 3, 4 or 6
5. Brain stem lesions
6. Cerebellar lesions
7. Vestibular lesions
8. High cervical cord lesions
9. Idiopathic or congenital

FURTHER READING

Harrison M J G 1981 British Journal of Hospital Medicine 26: 484

Some causes of 'giddiness'
1. True vertigo (q.v.)
2. Hypotension or hypertension
3. Anaemia
4. Intra-cranial hypertension
5. Hypoglycaemia
6. Epileptic aura
7. Migraine
8. Psychogenic

Causes of vertigo
1. Vestibular lesions
    (i) Physiological
    (ii) Labyrinthitis
    (iii) Menière's
    (iv) Drugs, e.g. quinine, salicylates
    (v) Otitis media
    (vi) Motion sickness
    (vii) 'Benign post-traumatic positional vertigo'
2. Vestibular nerve lesions
    (i) Acoustic neuroma
    (ii) Drugs, e.g. streptomycin
    (iii) Vestibular neuronitis
3. Brain stem, cerebellar or temporal lobe lesions
    (i) Pontine infarction or haemorrhage
    (ii) Vertebro-basilar insufficiency
    (iii) Basilar artery migraine
    (iv) Disseminated sclerosis
    (v) Tumours
    (vi) Syringobulbia
    (vii) Temporal lobe epilepsy

BASAL ARTERIES OF THE BRAIN

Anatomy

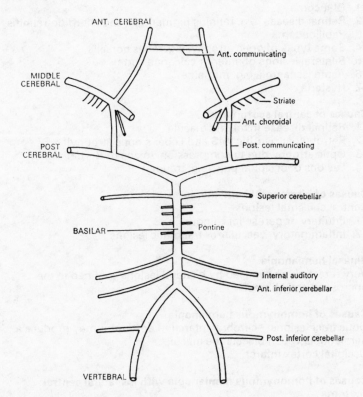

ANT. CEREBRAL

Ant. communicating

MIDDLE
CEREBRAL

Striate

Ant. choroidal

POST
CEREBRAL

Post. communicating

Superior cerebellar

BASILAR

Pontine

Internal auditory

Ant. inferior cerebellar

Post. inferior cerebellar

VERTEBRAL

Features of post. inf. cerebellar artery thrombosis
1. Sudden onset of severe vertigo
2. Ipsilateral cerebellar ataxia, with nystagmus to side of lesion
3. Contralateral sensory loss of trunk and limbs to pain and
   temperature
4. Ipsilateral involvement of 5th to 8th nerves
5. Bulbar palsy
6. Ipsilateral cervical sympathetic paralysis

PATTERNS OF VISUAL FIELD LOSS

Causes of concentric diminution ('tunnel vision')
1. Glaucoma
2. Retinal disease, e.g. retinitis pigmentosa and choroido-retinitis
3. Papilloedema
4. Some types of optic atrophy, e.g. tabes dorsalis
5. Bilateral lesions of anterior calcarine cortex
6. Acute ischaemia e.g. migraine
7. Hysteria

Causes of central scotoma
1. Retinal disease involving macula
2. Retrobulbar neuritis (MS and Leber's optic atrophy)
3. Optic atrophy due to compression, toxins or B_{12} deficiency
4. Lesions of occipital pole (e.g. trauma)

Causes of bitemporal hemianopia
Central chiasmal lesions
1. Pituitary or peri-sellar tumour
2. Inflammatory, vascular or traumatic lesions

Binasal hemianopia
Very rare, being produced by bilateral lesions confined to the uncrossed optic fibres

Causes of homonymous hemianopia
Optic tract lesions—cerebral infarction or tumour may produce a hemianopia which bisects the macula.
Occipital cortex infarct

Causes of homonymous hemianopia with ipsilateral central scotoma
Lesions of lateral part of optic chiasma which also affect the optic nerve
1. Pituitary tumour
2. Aneurysm of ant. communicating artery
3. Sphenoidal wing meningioma

Causes of homonymous quadrantanopia
Anteriorly placed lesions of the optic radiation, especially temporal lobe tumours. More posterior lesions of the optic radiation become more hemianopic

CAUSES OF OPTIC ATROPHY

1. *Glaucoma*
2. *Retinal lesions*
    Choroida-retinitis
    Intra-ocular haemorrhage, etc.
3. *Optic neuritis* (retrobulbar neuritis) (q.v.)
4. *Chronic papilloedema*
5. *Pressure on optic nerve*
    Tumour
    Aneurysm
    Paget's disease
6. *Division of optic nerve*
    Surgery
    Trauma

CAUSES OF OPTIC NEURITIS

1. *Ischaemia*, e.g. cranial arteritis
2. *Demyelinating disease*
    Multiple sclerosis
    Leucodystrophies
3. *Infective*
    Local: retinitis, periostitis, meningitis
    Systemic: syphilis, toxoplasmosis, typhoid fever
4. *Toxins*
    Methyl alcohol
    Lead
    Benzene
    Tobacco (defect in cyanide detoxication)
    Clioquinol (subacute myelo-optic neuropathy)
5. *Metabolic*
    Diabetes mellitus
    B_{12} deficiency
    Tropical ataxic neuropathy (cassava diet)
    Severe anaemia esp. haemorrhage
6. *Hereditary degenerations*
    e.g. Leber's, Friedreich's ataxia

FURTHER READING

McDonald W I 1977 British Journal of Hospital Medicine 18: 42
Perkin G D, Ross F C 1979 Optic neuritis and its differential diagnosis.
    Oxford Medical Publications, Oxford

CAUSES OF CATARACT

1. *Senility*
2. *Endocrine*
    Diabetes mellitus
    Hypoparathyroidism
    Corticosteroid therapy
    Cretinism
3. *Hereditary and congenital conditions*
    Rubella syndrome
    Atopic eczema
    Down's syndrome
    Hepatolenticular degeneration
    Galactosaemia
    Dystrophia myotonica
    Oculocerebrorenal syndrome (Lowe)
    Laurence-Moon-Biedl (retinitis pigmentosa, polydactyly, obesity, hypogonadism, mental retardation)
    Refsum's (retinitis pigmentosa, deafness, ataxia. neuropathy)
4. *Secondary to ocular disease*
    Glaucoma
    Ophthalmitis
    Degenerative myopia
    Retinal detachment
    Trauma
5. *Heat and irradiation*

CAUSES OF UVEITIS

(Uveal tract = iris, ciliary body and choroid)
1. *Miscellaneous systemic diseases*
    (i) Ankylosing spondylitis
    (ii) Reiter's disease
    (iii) Sarcoidosis
    (iv) Ulcerative colitis
    (v) Rheumatoid disease, esp. Still's
    (vi) Behcet's disease (esp. in Turkey and Japan)
2. *Infections*
    (i) Bacterial: TB
    (ii) Spirochaetal: Sy, relapsing fever, Weil's disease
    (iii) Fungal: Histoplasmosis (in USA)
    (iv) Protozoal: Malaria, toxoplasmosis
    (v) Nematode larvae: Toxocara of dog and cat
3. *Secondary to ocular disease*
    (i) Ophthalmitis
    (ii) Trauma
4. *Idiopathic*

FURTHER READING

Dinning W J 1980 British Journal of Hospital Medicine 24: 219

CAUSES OF PAPILLOEDEMA

1. *Raised intra-cranial pressure*
2. *Arterial hypertension*
3. *Optic neuritis* (papillitis)
4. *Obstructed retinal venous drainage*
    (i) tumour
    (ii) thrombosis of central retinal vein
    (iii) cavernous sinus thrombosis
5. *Miscellaneous rare causes*
    (i) Hypercapnia
    (ii) Exophthalmos
    (iii) SABE
    (iv) Hypoparathyroidism
    (v) Sudden or severe anaemia
    (vi) Vit. A poisoning
    (vii) Lead poisoning

Papilloedema without papillitis tends to produce a large blind spot but normal visual acuity

Papillitis (Retrobulbar neuritis) tends to produce a large central scotoma with poor visual acuity, and pain on eye movement

CERVICAL SYMPATHETIC PATHWAY TO THE EYE

1. Mid-brain (superior colliculus)
2. Tecto-spinal tract (adjacent to lateral spino-thalamic tract)
3. C8, T1 and 2 ventral roots
4. Cervical sympathetic trunk
5. Internal carotid and cavernous nerve plexus
6. Ophthalmic division of the trigeminal nerve

CAUSES OF PTOSIS

1. Congenital
2. Oculomotor nerve lesion
3. Cervical sympathetic lesion (Horner's)
4. Myasthenia gravis
5. Myopathy
6. Tabes dorsalis
7. Hysteria

Exclude congenital microphthalmos, contralateral exophthalmos

CAUSES OF MYDRIASIS (abnormally large pupil)

1. *Oculomotor nerve lesions*
   Characterized by
   (i) Marked ptosis
   (ii) Large regular pupil fixed to light and accommodation
   (iii) External ophthalmoplegia (eye looks down and out)
2. *Parasympathetic paralysis*, e.g. atropine (acts via oculomotor nerve)
3. *Sympathetic stimulation* (e.g. adrenaline or cocaine)
   Pupils reacts normally to light and accommodation
4. *Optic nerve lesion*
   Pupil reacts sluggishly to direct light, but normally to consensual light and accommodation
5. *Lesions of eye* such as iritis, cataract or vitreous haemorrhage
6. *Deep coma*
7. *Myotonic pupil* (Holmes-Adie)

EYE MOVEMENTS

With the eye turned *laterally* the *elevators* and depressors are the *superior* and inferior recti respectively
With the eye turned *medially* the *elevators* and depressors are the *inferior* and superior obliques respectively

CAUSES OF TRANSIENT FOCAL CEREBRAL ISCHAEMIC ATTACKS (TIA)

1. Emboli from heart or neck vessels
2. Mechanical effects
   (i) Cervical spondylosis
   (ii) Subclavian steal (proximal subclavian stenosis)
   (iii) Shunts
3. Increased arterial resistance, e.g. hypertension or migraine
4. Hypotension
5. Increased blood viscosity, e.g. polycythaemia
6. Anaemia

FURTHER READING

Harrison M J G 1974 In: Ledingham J G G (ed) Advanced medicine, symposium 10. Pitman, London, p 215

CAUSES OF RETINAL HAEMORRHAGE

1. Diabetes mellitus
2. Hypertension
3. Raised IC pressure
4. Retinal vein thrombosis
5. Trauma and retinal detachment
6. Arteritis (PN, cranial arteritis, etc.)
7. Sub-arachnoid haemorrhage
8. Severe anaemia, especially PA
9. Bleeding diathesis—defect in platelets (esp. leukaemia), vessels or coagulation factors

CAUSES OF SUDDEN BLINDNESS

1. Trauma—ocular or post-head injury
2. Vitreous haemorrhage, especially in diabetics
3. Retinal detachment
4. Acute glaucoma
5. Embolism or spasm of retinal artery
6. Thrombosis of retinal vein
7. Acute optic neuritis, esp. cranial arteritis and methyl alcohol poisoning
8. Cerebral infarct or haemorrhage
9. Hypertensive encephalopathy
10. Migraine
11. Acute hydrocephalus, esp. in children
12. Transient 'blackout', e.g. vasovagal
13. Welding lights etc.
14. Hysteria

DRUG-INDUCED EYE DISEASE

1. **Eyelids**
   Pigmentation—chlorpromazine
   Eczema—topical chloramphenicol
   Angio-oedema—penicillin

2. **Conjunctiva and cornea**
   Punctate deposits—chloroquine, chlorpromazine
   Stevens-Johnson syndrome—sulphonamides
   Oculo-mucocutaneous syndrome—practolol

3. **Uvea** (iris, ciliary body and choroid)
   Blurred vision—anticholinergics
   Glaucoma—anticholinergics, antihistamines, antiparkinsonian drugs

4. Lens

Transient myopia—tetracycline, sulphonamide, acetazolamide
Cataract—cholinesterase inhibitors, glucocorticoids,
    phenothiazines

5. Retina

Retinopathy—chloroquine and derivatives
    phenothiazines, esp. thioridazine

6. Optic nerve

Neuropathy
(i) Neurotoxic—antituberculous drugs (isoniazid,
 streptomycin, ethambutol)
(ii) Ischaemic—quinine
(iii) Nutritional—penicillamine (pyridoxine deficiency)

FURTHER READING

Davison S I 1980 British Journal of Hospital Medicine 24: 24

SPINAL CORD

Transverse section

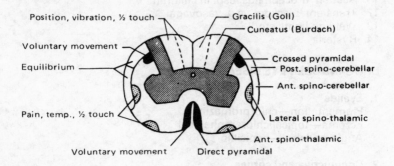

Position, vibration, ½ touch — Gracilis (Goll)
— Cuneatus (Burdach)
Voluntary movement
Equilibrium — Crossed pyramidal
Post. spino-cerebellar
Ant. spino-cerebellar
Pain, temp., ½ touch — Lateral spino-thalamic
— Ant. spino-thalamic
Voluntary movement   Direct pyramidal

Tendon Reflexes		Superficial Reflexes	
Ankle	S 1, 2	Cremasteric	L 1, 2
Knee	L 3, 4	Anal	S 3, 4
Biceps	C 5	Plantar	S1
Supinator	C 5, 6	Abdominal	T 8 to 12
Triceps	C 7		

Nerve supply of diaphram
Phrenic n. (C 3, 4, 5) descends under cover of sternomastiod m., passes in front of subclavian artery, then descends vertically in front of root of lung and passes between pericardium and mediastinal pleura to diaphragm. The diaphragm is also innervated peripherally by the lower 7 intercostal nerves.

Course of recurrent laryngeal nerves
Right R.L.N. arises from vagus in the neck and winds backwards round first part of R. subclavian artery. *Left* R.L.N. arises from vagus in the superior mediastinum and winds backwards round arch of aorta. Both nerves then ascend between trachea and oesophagus and supply all muscles of larynx except cricothyroid.

   Bilateral paralysis causes stridor ('cadaveric' cords).
   Unilateral paralysis causes dysphonia with 'bovine' cough.

Causes of cord compression
1. *Vertebral*
   (i) Congenital bony anomaly
   (ii) Trauma
   (iii) Vertebral collapse
   (iv) Disc prolapse, spondylolisthesis, spondylosis
   (v) Neoplasm (primary or secondary)
   (vi) Paget's
   (vii) Infection—TB or pyogenic
2. *Extra-dural*
   (i) Hodgkin's, leukaemic infiltrate or metastases
   (ii) Abscess
   (iii) Cyst
3. *Intra-dural extra-medullary*
   (i) Neoplasm (meningioma, neurofibroma)
   (ii) Arachnoiditis
   (iii) Arachnoid cyst
4. *Intra-medullary*
   (i) Neoplasm, esp. glioma
   (ii) Cyst or syringomyelia
   (iii) Haematomyelia

FURTHER READING

Uttley D 1981 British Journal of Hospital Medicine 26: 607

Causes of paraplegia
1. Hereditary spastic paraplegia
2. Cerebral birth injury
3. Trauma
4. Cord compression—intra- or extra-medullary (q.v.)
5. Multiple sclerosis
6. Transverse myelitis
7. Spinal artery occlusion, including meningo-vascular Sy.
8. Syringomyelia
9. Motor neurone disease
10. Poliomyelitis
11. Sub-acute combined degeneration
12. Guillain-Barré (Landry's ascending paralysis)
13. Friedreich's ataxia; familial spastic paraplegia, etc.
14. Sagittal sinus thrombosis
15. Midline pre-central meningioma
16. Hysteria

Causes of dissociated anaesthesia (Loss of pain and temperature, but preservation of other sensation)
1. *Central cord lesion* affecting the crossing fibres e.g. syringomyelia
2. *Cord hemisection* (*Brown-Sequard*)
   e.g. compression or intramedullary neoplasm
   Features
   (i) L.M.N. lesion at level of lesion
   (ii) U.M.N. lesion below level of lesion
   (iii) Ipsilateral loss of position, vibration and touch
   (iv) Contralateral loss of pain and temperature
3. *Lesions of lateral medulla*
   e.g. posterior-inferior cerebellar thrombosis or syringobulbia

PERIPHERAL NERVES

Nerve supply to muscles of front of forearm

Ulnar nerve supplies
1. Flexor carpi ulnaris
2. Half of flexor digitorum profundus

Median nerve supplies all the rest

Nerve supply to short muscles of hand
Median nerve supplies
1. Lateral two lumbricals
2. Opponens pollicis
3. Abductor pollicis brevis
4. Flexor pollicis brevis
Mnemonic—'LOAF'

Ulnar nerve supplies all the rest
Abductor pollicis brevis is paralysed in T1 root lesions but not in
ulnar nerve lesions

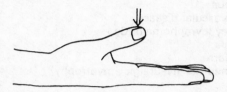

To test abductor pollicis brevis the thumb is moved vertically against
resistance, with the hand supine

Causes of wasting of small muscles of hand
1. Cord lesions at T1 level
    Motor neurone disease
    Tumour
    Syringomyelia
    Meningo-vascular Sy.
    Cord compression (p. 121)
2. Root lesions
    Cervical spondylosis
    Neurofibroma, etc.
3. Brachial plexus lesions
    Klumpke paralysis
    Cervical rib, etc.
4. Ulnar or median nerve lesions
5. Arthritis of hand or wrist, or disuse atrophy

Causes of peripheral neuropathy
1. *Idiopathic*
2. *Metabolic*
    Diabetes mellitus
    Amyloidosis
    Acute intermittent porphyria
    Chronic uraemia
    Dysproteinaemia
3. *Vitamin deficiency*
    Subacute combined degeneration (B_{12})
    B complex (alcoholism, beri-beri)
    Pellagra
4. *Infection*
    Diphtheria
    Leprosy
    Tetanus
    Botulism

(contd)

5. *Drugs and Chemicals*
   Isoniazid, nitrofurantoin, vincristine
   Heavy metals (Pb, Hg)
   Organic chemicals, e.g. triorthocresyl phosphate
6. *Miscellaneous*
   Collagen-vascular disease
   Malignancy (Lymphoma or Ca.)
   Sarcoidosis
   Guillain-Barré
   'Brachial neuritis' (Neuralgic amyotrophy)
7. *Mechanical*
   Trauma, compression, stretching
8. *Hereditary*
   Hereditary ataxias
   Hereditary sensory radicular neuropathy (Denny-Brown)
   Hypertrophic interstitial neuritis (Déjerine-Sottas)
   Peroneal muscular atrophy (Charcot-Marie-Tooth)
   Refsum's disease

FURTHER READING

Hughes R A C 1978 British Journal of Hospital Medicine 20: 688

Causes of mononeuritis multiplex
1. Polyarteritis nodosa
2. Diabetes mellitus
3. Leprosy
4. Carcinoma
5. Sarcoidosis
6. Rheumatoid disease

Types of non-metastatic carcinomatous neuromyopathy
1. *Encephalopathy*
   (i) Progressive multifocal leukoencephalopathy
   (ii) Polio-encephalopathy
   (iii) Cerebellar degeneration
   (iv) Dementia
2. *Encephalomyelitis*
3. *Neuropathy*
   Motor, sensory or mixed
4. *Neuromuscular disorder*
   (i) Myasthenia gravis
   (ii) Eaton Lambert syndrome (weakness which improves with tetanic stimulation)
5. *Dermatomyositis or polymyositis*
6. *Non-specific muscle wasting*
7. *Neuromyotonia*
8. *Muscle weakness due to ectopic hormones,* e.g. ACTH or parathormone

FURTHER READING

Croft P 1977 British Journal of Hospital Medicine 17: 356

Dermatomes in the upper limb

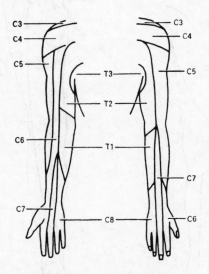

CLINICAL VARIETIES OF NEURO-SYPHILIS

1. Asymptomatic; Argyll Robertson pupils may be the only sign
2. Meningitis
   (i) Acute
   (ii) Chronic pachymeningitis
3. Vascular
   (i) Endarteritis of middle cerebral artery
   (ii) Endarteritis of anterior spinal artery (Erb's paraplegia)
4. GPI
5. Tabes dorsalis
6. Optic atrophy
7. Gumma of brain

FURTHER READING

Catterall R D 1977 British Journal of Hospital Medicine 17: 585

Dermatomes in the lower limb

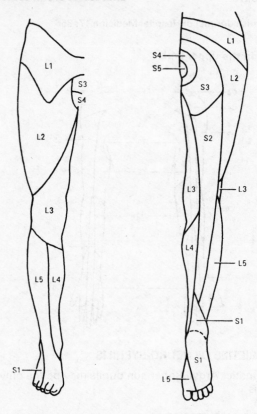

Dermatomes of head and neck

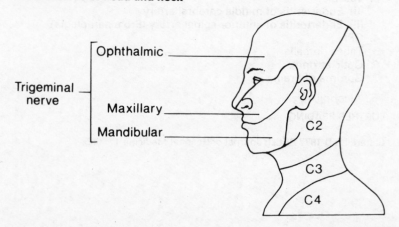

Causes of absent knee and ankle jerks with an extensor plantar response
1. Sub-acute combined degeneration
2. Syphilitic tabo-paresis
3. Friedreich's ataxia
4. Motor neurone disease
5. Diabetes mellitus
6. Conus medullaris lesion

ARGYLL ROBERTSON PUPILS (ACCOMMODATION REFLEX PRESENT)

The light reflex is interrupted between the lateral geniculate body and the oculomotor nucleus (probably in the pre-tectal area)

Causes
1. Syphilis, esp. tabes dorsalis
2. Diabetes mellitus
3. Rarely alcoholism, encephalitis, MS or vascular or neoplastic lesions of midbrain

CAUSES OF A CHARCOT JOINT

1. Tabes dorsalis
2. Syringomyelia
3. Diabetes mellitus
Rarely:
4. Cord lesion, e.g. trauma, meningomyelocoele, SACD
5. Leprosy, yaws
6. Congenital neuropathy (p. 124)
7. Congenital indifference to pain
8. Familial dysautonomia (Riley-Day)
9. Repeated intra-articular steroid injection

CAUSES OF TREMOR

1. Parkinsonism (p. 128)
2. Cerebellar lesion
3. Anxiety
4. Thyrotoxicosis
5. Alcoholism
6. Drugs e.g. tricyclic antidepressants
7. Heavy metals (e.g. 'hatters' shakes' due to mercury)
8. Neurosyphilis
9. Benign essential or familial tremor

CAUSES OF PARKINSONISM

(Tremor, rigidity and hypokinesia)
1. Idiopathic 'paralysis agitans'
2. Drugs—phenothiazines
        haloperidol
        reserpine
        methyldopa
        tetrabenazine
3. Toxins—manganese
        carbon monoxide
        kernicterus
4. Post-encephalitic
5. Repeated head injury
6. Rarely syphilis, cerebral tumour, hypoparathyroidism or Behcet's

Parkinsonian features also occur in
1. Phenylketonuria
2. Hepatolenticular degeneration
3. Shy-Drager syndrome (with autonomic dysfunction)
4. Progressive supranuclear palsy with paralysis of conjugate gaze (Steele-Richardson syndrome)
5. Creutzfeld-Jakob transmissible dementia
6. Olivopontocerebellar atrophy

Atheroma as a cause of parkinsonism is disputed

FURTHER READING

Lenman J A R 1982 Hospital Update 8: 11

CAUSES OF DISORDERED NEUROMUSCULAR TRANSMISSION

1. *Hereditary*
    (i) Hereditary myasthenia gravis
    (ii) Pseudocholinesterase deficiency (suxamethonium paralysis)
2. *Drugs and toxins*
    (i) Depolarizing drugs
    (ii) Anticholinesterase poisons (e.g. 'nerve gas')
    (iii) Botulism
    (iv) Venom of Black Widow spider, puff-fish, etc.
    (v) Magnesium poisoning
    (vi) Antibiotics, especially kanamycin
3. *Idiopathic myasthenia gravis*
    (possibly auto-immune)
4. *Myasthenia associated with other disease*
    (i) Thyrotoxicosis
    (ii) Malignancy (Eaton Lambert syndrome)
    (iii) SLE or polymyositis

FURTHER READING

Simpson J A 1974 In: Walton J N (ed) Disorders of voluntary muscle, 3rd edn. Churchill Livingstone, Edinburgh, p 653

MYOTONIA

1. *Myotonia congenita*
   Thomson: Dominant
   Becker: Recessive, more severe and later onset
2. *Dystrophia myotonica*
   (i) Myotonia and muscle atrophy
   (ii) Characteristic facies with ptosis and frontal baldness
   (iii) Cataracts, gonadal atrophy, heart disease, hypoventilation, bone changes and dementia
3. *Paramyotonia congenita*
   Myotonia and weakness induced by cold, sometimes with fluctuation in serum potassium

FURTHER READING

Walton J N, Gardner-Medwin D 1974 In: Walton J N (ed) Disorders of voluntary muscle, 3rd edn. Churchill Livingstones Edinburgh, p 592
Gardner-Medwin D 1977 British Journal of Hospital Medicine 17: 314

CONGENITAL MYOPATHIES

   (i) Benign congenital hypotonia
   (ii) Central core disease
   (iii) Nemaline myopathy
   (iv) Myotubular myopathy
   (v) Congenital universal muscular hypoplasia
   (vi) Mitochondrial defects, e.g. megaconial myopathy
   (vii) Arthrogryphosis multiplex congenita

METABOLIC AND ENDOCRINE MYOPATHIES

1. *Periodic paralysis*
   Se K may fall, rise or remain constant during attacks
2. *Glycogen storage diseases* (p. 131)
3. *Mitochondrial overactivity*
   (i) Hypermetabolic myopathy
   (ii) Malignant hyperpyrexia during anaesthesia
4. *Nutritional myopathy*
   (i) Kwashiorkor
   (ii) Vitamin E deficiency

(contd)

5. *Drugs*
    (i) Glucocorticoids, especially triamcinolone
    (ii) Alcohol (p. 105)
    (iii) Drugs which induce hypokalaemia
    (iv) Heroin, amphetamine addiction
    (v) Chloroquine
    (vi) Vincristine
6. *Endocrine*
    (i) Hyper- or hypo-thyroidism
    (ii) Osteomalacia
    (iii) Acromegaly
    (iv) Cushing's syndrome
    (v) Hypoadrenalism
    (vi) Primary aldosteronism

FURTHER READING

Gardner-Medwin D 1977 British Journal of Hospital Medicine 17: 314
Mastaglia F L 1980 British Journal of Hospital Medicine 24: 8
McArdle B 1974 In: Walton J N (ed) Disorders of voluntary muscle, 3rd edn.
  Churchill Livingstone, Edinburgh, p 721

Causes of painful myopathy
1. Inflammatory
    (i) Polymyositis—dermatomyositis group
    (ii) Viral polymyositis
    (iii) Parasitic (trichinelliasis, cysticercosis)
2. Polymyalgia rheumatica
3. Acute alcoholic myopathy
4. Drug-induced
    (i) Due to hypokalaemia, e.g. diuretics, purgatives
    (ii) Mechanism unknown, e.g. heroin, amphetamine
5. Associated with osteomalacia
6. Specific defects in muscle energy metabolism, e.g. deficiency
   of myophosphorylase, phosphofructokinase etc.
7. Idiopathic paroxysmal myoglobinurias
8. Idiopathic

FURTHER READING

Morgan-Hughes J A 1979 British Journal of Hospital Medicine 22: 360

GLYCOGEN STORAGE DISEASES

TYPE I

Glucose-6-phosphatase deficiency (von Gierke). Hepatomegaly, retarded growth, hypoglycaemia, acidosis and ketonuria

TYPE II

1–4 Glucosidase deficiency (Pompe). Dyspnoea, cardiomegaly and weak hypotonic muscles.

TYPE III
Amylo-1–6-glucosidase deficiency (Cori). Clinically resembles Type I, but milder, with no hypoglycaemia.

TYPE IV

Amylo-transglucosidase deficiency (Anderson). Cirrhosis and death in early childhood. Very rare.

TYPE V

Muscle phosphorylase deficiency (McArdle). Pain, weakness and stiffness during exercise.

TYPE VI

(Her). Heterogeneous group with hepatomegaly and retarded growth.
Several other rare types exist.

FURTHER READING

McArdle B 1974 In: Walton J N (ed) Disorders of voluntary muscle, 3rd edn. Churchill Livingstone, Edinburgh, p 734

PROGRESSIVE MUSCULAR DYSTROPHIES

1. *X linked recessive* (*'Pseudo-hypertrophic'*)
   (i) Duchenne (severe)
   (ii) Becker (milder and of later onset)
2. *Autosomal recessive*
   Limb girdle type (Erb)
3. *Autosomal dominant*
   (i) Facio-scapulo-humeral (Landouzy and Déjerine)
   (ii) Distal myopathy of late onset (Welander)
   (iii) Ocular myopathy (may also be either retinopathy or dysphagia)

Certain exceptions occur to this simple genetic classification

FURTHER READING

Walton J N, Gardner-Medwin D 1974 In: Walton J N (ed) Disorders of voluntary muscle, 3rd edn. Churchill Livingstone, Edinburgh, p 561

FOUR SIMILAR SIGNS

1. *Kernig's sign.* To detect meningeal irritation

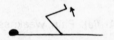

Straightening leg with hip flexed produces pain and spasm of hamstrings

2. *Brudzinski's sign.* To detect meningeal irritation

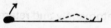

Flexing neck produces flexion of lower limbs

3. *Thomas's test.* To detect fixed flexion deformity of the hip-joint

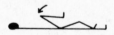

Eliminating lumbar lordosis produces flexion of the affected hip

4. *Straight-leg raising test.* To detect lesions of sciatic nerve or its spinal roots

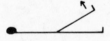

Straight-leg raising produces pain below the normal full excursion

Endocrine and bone disease

DIABETES MELLITUS

Definition. Diabetes mellitus is a syndrome which merges with the normal, and diagnostic criteria are therefore arbitrary.

The definition used by the British Diabetic Association depends on the oral glucose tolerance test. The test indicates diabetes if, after a 50 g glucose load, the venous blood concentration is 7 mmol/l (120 mg/100 ml) or more at 2 h and 9 mmol /l (160 mg/100 ml) or more at some other time during the test.

Microvascular complications tend to develop only in subjects whose 2 hr value exceeds 11 mmol/l, and a more liberal definition has been suggested:

Definite D M: Fasting level over 7 mmol/l, and over 10 mmol/l at 2 hr

Impaired Glucose Tolerance: Fasting level under 7 mmol/l, but over 7 mmol/l at 2 hr Many patients in this group will spontaneously revert to a normal GTT

FURTHER READING

Keen H 1981 Medicine International 1: 327
Keen H, Jarrett J 1978 Medicine, 3rd, series 11: 517
Sönksen P H, Brown P M 1981 In: Dawson A M, Compston N, Besser G M (eds) Recent advances in medicine—18. Churchill Livingstone, Edinburgh, p 315

Causes of diabetes mellitus
1. *Idiopathic*
    (i) Subclinical—Impaired glucose tolerance
    (ii) Clinical—Insulin dependent ('juvenile onset')
            Non-insulin dependent ('maturity onset')
2. *Secondary to other disease*
    (i) Pancreatic disease (pancreatitis, Ca., haemochromatosis, etc.)
    (ii) Cushing's syndrome

(*contd*)

(iii) Acromegaly
(iv) Phaeochromocytoma
 (v) Cirrhosis
(vi) Chronic renal failure
3. *Drugs*
   (i) Glucocorticoids
  (ii) Thiazides
 (iii) Oral contraceptives
  (iv) Diazoxide

FURTHER READING

Cudworth A G 1976 British Journal of Hospital Medicine 15: 207
Keen H, Jarrett J 1978 Medicine, 3rd series, 11: 517

Chronic complications of diabetes mellitus
1. *Ocular*
   (i) Blurred vision due to fluctuations in blood sugar
  (ii) Cataracts
 (iii) Retinopathy:
       Venous engorgement
       Capillary microaneurysms
       'Blot' haemorrhages
       'Waxy' exudates
       Retinal infarcts ('cottonwool spots')
       Vitreous haemorrhage
       Retinitis proliferans
       Retinal detachment
  (iv) Rubeosis iridis (new blood vessels over iris)—may cause
       glaucoma
2. *Neurological*
   (i) Cerebral disturbance due to hyper- or hypoglycaemia
  (ii) Cerebral lesions due to atheroma
 (iii) Peripheral neuropathy
       a. Asymptomatic loss of ankle-jerks and vibration sense
       b. Painful subacute neuritis, usually in lower limbs
       c. Mononeuritis multiplex (often asymmetrical)
       d. Isolated cranial nerve lesions
       e. Autonomic neuropathy
  (iv) Diabetic pseudo-tabes
   (v) Diabetic amyotrophy
  (vi) 'Insulin neuritis' during stabilisation
3. *Renal*
   (i) Pyelonephritis, sometimes with papillary necrosis.
  (ii) Glomerulonephritis
       a. Kimmelstiel-Wilson (eosinophilic nodules in glomerular
          tuft)
       b. Proliferative, with sclerosed basement membrane
 (iii) Atherosclerosis and hypertensive vascular changes

4. *Vascular*
   Occlusion of large vessels (atheroma) or small vessels
   (endarteritis) may cause ischaemia of feet, myocardium, brain
   or kidneys
5. *Dermatological*
   (i) Fat atrophy or hypertrophy or fibrosis at insulin injection
       sites
   (ii) Ulcers due to neuropathy or ischaemia
   (iii) Infections, especially furuncles and Candidosis
   (iv) Pigmented scars over shins ('diabetic dermopathy')
   (v) Xanthomata
   (vi) Necrobiosis lipoidica
   (vii) Widespread granuloma annulare
6. *Systemic infections*
   Incidence of TB, chronic urinary infections and deep mycoses is
   increased

FURTHER READING

Keen H, Jarrett J 1978 Medicine, 3rd series, 11: 525
Kohner E M, Watkins P J, Keen H 1981 Medicine International 1: 343

DIABETES AND PREGNANCY

Pregnancy produces a tendency to both keto-acidosis and fasting
hypoglycaemia. This paradox is due to
  1. Counteraction of maternal insulin by placental hormones
  2. Removal of glucose by the fetus

COMPLICATIONS OF PREGNANCY IN THE DIABETIC

1. *Maternal morbidity*
   (i) Hydramnios
   (ii) Pre-eclampsia
   (iii) Pregnancy probably accelerates diabetic micro-angiopathy
         and some authors recommend abortion and sterilization in
         women with proliferative retinopathy or nephropathy
2. *Fetal mortality* Still-birth (5 – 10%) or neonatal death (5 – 10%)
   due to
   (i) Hyaline membrane disease (preterm delivery)
   (ii) Congenital anomalies (often cardiac or neurological)
3. *Fetal morbidity*
   (i) Macrosomia (excessive size)
   (ii) Hypoglycaemia
   (iii) Congenital anomalies
   (iv) Respiratory distress (due to pre-term delivery)
   (v) Hypocalcaemia (maternal hypercalcaemia suppresses the
       fetal parathyroid)

FURTHER READING

Burrows G N, Ferris T F 1975 Medical complications during pregnancy.
  Saunders, Philadelphia, p 170
Essex Nina 1976 British Journal of Hospital Medicine 15: 333

CAUSES OF HYPOGLYCAEMIA

1. *Starvation and exercise*
2. *Reaction to glucose ingestion*
      Functional
      Early diabetes mellitus
      Post-gastrectomy
3. *β-cell overactivity*
      Insulinoma
      Hyperplasia
4. *Endocrine disease*
      Hypothyroidism
      Hypopituitarism
      Hypoadrenalism
5. *Drugs*
      Insulin
      Sulphonylureas
      Salicylates
      Paracetamol
      Ackee, etc.
6. *Sensitivity to:*
      Leucine
      Galactose, fructose
      Alcohol, tobacco
7. *Liver disease*
      Glycogen storage disease
      Hepatoma
8. *Neoplasm*
      Especially large fibrosarcoma
9. *In infancy*
      (i) Idiopathic hypoglycaemia of infancy
      (ii) After fetal malnutrition

FURTHER READING

Marks V 1975 Medicine, 2nd series, 14: 646
Turner R, Rubenstein A H, Foster D W 1981 Medicine International 1: 351

CONGENITAL ADRENAL HYPERPLASIA

Cortisol, aldosterone and androgen synthesis may be affected depending on site of enzyme block.

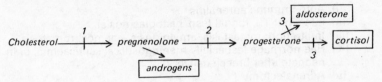

Site 1

Lipoid hyperplasia (20–22 desmolase deficiency). Very rare
Severe deficiency in all 3 hormones
Adrenal cortex filled with lipid

Site 2

3β-hydroxysteroid dehydrogenase defect. Very rare
Androgens unaffected

Site 3

21-hydroxylase defect
Clinical features
  (i)   Ambiguous genitalia
  (ii) Virilization in female, precocious pseudo-puberty in male
  (iii) Electrolyte imbalance
  (iv) Rapid growth, but eventual short stature.
The plasma 17-hydroxyprogesterone is increased.

Site 3

11β-hydroxylase defect
Hypertension with virilization

Rarer syndromes also exist

FURTHER READING

Anderson D C et al 1981 Hospital Update 7: 1205
Bailey J D et al 1978 Medicine, 3rd series, 10: 472

CAUSES OF ADRENAL INSUFFICIENCY

Primary
1. Acute or chronic gland destruction
   (i) Auto-immune adrenalitis
   (ii) Infection: TB, fungal (esp. histoplasmosis).
   (iii) Infiltration: metastasis, amyloidosis, haemochromatosis
   (iv) Haemorrhage (especially meningococcal septicaemia, or in neonate after breech delivery)
   (v) Adrenalectomy
   (vi) Adrenal vein thrombosis (e.g. after adrenal venography)
2. Metabolic failure
   (i) Virilizing hyperplasia, e.g. C21-hydroxylase deficiency
   (ii) Enzyme inhibitors, e.g. metyrapone
   (iii) Cytotoxic drugs, e.g. opDDD

Secondary
1. Hypopituitarism
2. Suppression of hypothalamic-pituitary axis
   (i) Exogenous glucocorticoids
   (ii) Endogenous glucocorticoids, e.g. Cushing's syndrome following tumour removal

FURTHER READING

Besser M 1978 Medicine, 3rd series, 9: 418
Hall R 1981 Medicine International 1: 276

RENIN, ANGIOTENSIN AND ALDOSTERONE

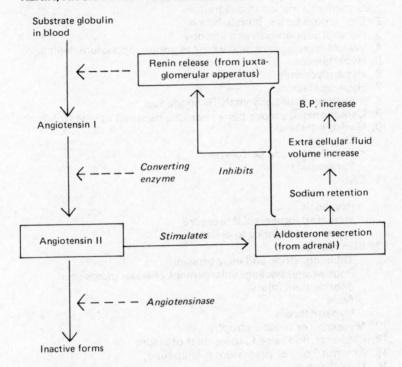

Saralasin competitively antagonises the acute pressor effect of angiotensin II
Captopril inhibits the enzyme that converts angiotensin I to angiotensin II.

FURTHER READING

Brown J J et al 1976 In: Peters D K (ed) Advanced medicine, symposium 12. Pitman, London, p 407
Hollenberg N K, Williams G H 1980 Advances in Internal Medicine vol 25, Year Book Medical Pub. Inc, Chicago, p 327–361
Vidt D G et al 1982 New England Journal of Medicine 306: 214

Hazards of systemic glucocorticoid therapy
1. Growth retardation in children
2. Cushingoid facies, buffalo hump
3. Adrenal suppression and atrophy
4. Weight gain, sodium and water retention, potassium depletion
5. Hypertension
6. Hyperglycaemia
7. Hyperlipidaemia
8. Infections, especially viral, TB and fungal
9. Osteoporosis, aseptic bone necrosis, ruptured Achilles tendon
10. Gastro-intestinal
    Dyspepsia
    Peptic ulcer and perforation
    Pancreatitis
11. CNS
    Euphoria
    Psychosis
    Increased intra-cranial pressure
    Increased tendency to epilepsy
12. Skin changes
    Thinning, striae and easy bruising
    Poor wound healing, enlargement of stasis ulcers or
    débridement injury
    Acne
    Hypertrichosis
13. Myopathy or muscle atrophy
14. Cataracts, and raised intra-ocular pressure
15. Amenorrhoea or premature menopause
16. Hypothermia
17. Withdrawal phenomena (vomiting, panniculitis,
    hypercalcaemia)
18. 'Rebound' of disease on reduction of dosage
19. Teratogenicity (fetal cleft palate)

FURTHER READING

Myles A B, Daly J R (eds) 1975 Corticosteroid and ACTH Treatment Arnold,
    London

CAUSES OF GYNAECOMASTIA

1. Hermaphroditism or pseudo-hermaphroditism (p. 145)
2. Endocrine
   Normal puberty and neonatal
   Hypothyroidism
   Thyrotoxicosis
   Hypoadrenalism
   Testicular atrophy
   Testicular and adrenal tumours
   Acromegaly
   Hypothalamic lesions
3. Cirrhosis
4. Carcinoma or lymphoma
5. Refeeding after malnutrition
6. Renal failure with dialysis
7. Paraplegia
8. Erythroderma
9. Leprosy
10. Drugs
    Sex hormones
    Spironolactone
    Amphetamine
    Reserpine
    Digitalis
    Methyldopa etc.

FURTHER READING

Anderson D C, Large D M 1978 Medicine, 3rd series, 10: 460

CAUSES OF GALACTORRHOEA

1. Physiological (post-partum and neonatal)
2. Prolactin-secreting pituitary tumour
3. Pituitary stalk or hypothalamic lesion
4. Ectopic prolactin production, e.g. bronchial Ca.
5. Drugs, e.g.
   Phenothiazines
   Oral contraceptives
   Haloperidol
   Tricyclic antidepressants
   Methyldopa
   Meprobamate
   Reserpine
6. Chest will injury (surgery, herpes zoster, mesothelioma)
   Probably stimulates neurological pathway of suckling reflex
7. Hysterectomy
8. Hypothyroidism

FURTHER READING

Turkington R W 1972 Advances in Internal Medicine 18: 363

CAUSES OF AMENORRHOEA

Physiological
1. Pre-pubertal
2. Pregnancy
3. Menopausal

Pathological
1. *Anatomical*
   (i) Uterine anomaly
   (ii) Hysterectomy
   (iii) Cryptomenorrhoea

2. *Hypothalamic-pituitary axis*
   (i) 'Functional' amenorrhoea: change in environment, emotional upset, rapid change in weight
   (ii) Severe systemic disease: e.g. TB
   (iii) Hyperprolactinaemia
   (iv) Hypopituitarism
   (v) Isolated gonadotrophin deficiency
   (vi) Thyrotoxicosis
   (vii) Drugs: oestrogen, progesterone, testosterone, glucocorticoids, spironolactone

3. *Primary ovarian disease*
    (i) Oophorectomy
    (ii) Irradiation or cytotoxic drugs
    (iii) Pelvic TB
    (iv) Auto-immune, e.g. associated with Addison's disease.
4. *Virilizing syndromes*
    (i) Genetic intersex (p. 145)
    (ii) Ovarian
        Stein-Leventhal syndrome (polycystic ovary)
        Virilizing tumours, e.g. androblastoma
    (iii) Adrenal
        Congenital adrenal hyperplasia
        Acquired virilizing adenoma or Ca
5. *Oestrogen or progesterone excess*
    (i) Follicular or lutein retention cyst
    (ii) Sex cord stromal tumours

FURTHER READING

Jacobs H S 1978 Medicine, 3rd series, 9: 443
Marshall J C 1981 Medicine, International 1: 291

PROSTAGLANDINS

Possible physiological roles for prostaglandins
1. Reproduction
    (i) Luteolysis
    (ii) Transport of sperm and ova
    (iii) Induction of labour
    (iv) Patency of ductus arteriosus
2. Neurological
    (i) Feedback inhibition of neurotransmission
    (ii) Enhancement of pain and pruritus
    (iii) Control of body temperature
3. Control of arterial blood pressure
4. Control of platelet aggregation
5. Inhibition of gastric acid secretion
6. Renal autoregulation

FURTHER READING

Hillier K 1980 Prescribers' Journal 20: 142
Pike J E 1976 Journal of Investigative Dermatology 67: 650

BIOSYNTHESIS OF PROSTAGLANDINS

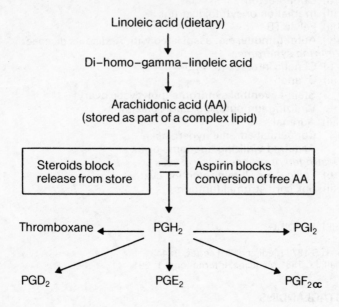

Linoleic acid (dietary)

↓

Di–homo–gamma–linoleic acid

↓

Arachidonic acid (AA)
(stored as part of a complex lipid)

| Steroids block release from store | Aspirin blocks conversion of free AA |

Thromboxane ← PGH_2 → PGI_2

PGD_2 PGE_2 $PGF_{2\alpha}$

FURTHER READING

Horton E W 1979 British Journal of Hospital Medicine 21: 260

CAUSES OF PRECOCIOUS PUBERTY

A. **True precocity** (premature activation of pituitary—hypothalamic axis)
  1. *Constitutional* (usually female, may be familial)
  2. *Secondary*
      (i) Tumours near the hypothalamus, e.g. pinealoma, hamartoma, teratoma etc.
      (ii) Brain damage, e.g. encephalitis, hydrocephalus, etc.
      (iii) Polyostotic fibrous dysplasia (Albright's syndrome)
      (iv) Hepatic cell carcinoma

B. Pseudo-precocity (secondary sexual development with immature gonads)

Overproduction of androgen or oestrogen by
  (i) Disease of ovary, testis or adrenal
  (ii) Teratoma
  (iii) Exogenous hormone

FURTHER READING

Brook C G D 1981 Medicine International 1: 315

INTERSEXUAL STATES

True hermaphrodites have both testicular and ovarian elements in the gonads

Male pseudo-hermaphrodites have testes but are feminized

Female pseudo-hermaphrodites have ovaries but are virilised

Causes
  1. *Genetic*
      (i) Turner's: XO
      (ii) Chromatin positive ovarian dysgenesis
          Abnormal X
          Mosaics
      (iii) Klinefelter's: XXY
      (iv) 'Super-females': XXX, etc.
      (v) 'Super-males': XYY, etc.
      (vi) Mosaics: XY/XO, XX/XY, etc.
      (vii) Gonadal dysgenesis: female phenotype
  2. *Hormonal*
Female
      (i) Congenital adrenal hyperplasia
      (ii) Virilising tumour of mother during pregnancy
      (iii) Sex hormones given to mother during pregnancy, e.g. to prevent abortion
Male
          End-organ unresponsiveness to androgens

FURTHER READING

Sizonenko P C, Theintz G E 1981 Medicine International 1: 319

THE THYROID

CAUSES OF HYPOTHYROIDISM

A. Primary (thyroid gland failure)
  1. Congenital
      (i) Absence or maldevelopment of thyroid gland
      (ii) Endemic cretinism (maternal iodine deficiency)
      (iii) Dyshormonogenesis (enzyme defects affect hormone synthesis)
            e.g. peroxidase deficiency
  2. Auto-immune thyroiditis
  3. Iatrogenic
      (i) Surgery
      (ii) Irradiation
      (iii) Anti-thyroid drugs
  4. Dietary iodine deficiency
  5. Acquired enzyme defects due to goitrogens (dietary or drugs)
  6. Riedel's thyroiditis (very rare)

B. Secondary (TSH deficiency)
  1. Hypopituitarism
  2. Rarely hypothalamic lesion (TRH deficiency)

CAUSES OF HYPERTHYROIDISM

  1. Graves' disease and toxic multinodular goitre
  2. Toxic adenoma
  3. Iatrogens
      (i) Overdosage with thyroid hormone
      (ii) Following administration of iodine to goitrous patient (Jod-Basedow phenomenon)
  4. Transient, associated with thyroiditis
  5. Ectopic TSH secretion by neoplasm, e.g. choriocarcinoma
  6. Ectopic thyroid secretion by struma ovarii

FURTHER READING

Hoffenberg R 1981 Medicine International 1: 256

CAUSES OF PROPTOSIS

1. *Dysthyroid exophthalmos*, usually with lid retraction, lid lag and weak upward gaze
   CAT scan shows enlarged extraocular muscles, and TRH test shows abnormal TSH response
2. *Neoplasm*
   (i) Benign, e.g. dermoid
   (ii) Malignant primary or secondary
3. *Vascular*, e.g. capillary haemangioma
4. *Bony malformation*
5. *Inflammation*, e.g. pseudotumour, cellulitis.
6. *Systemic disease*, e.g. Wegener's, histiocytosis X, xanthogranuloma, sarcoidosis

FURTHER READING

Henk J M 1981 Hospital Update 7: 439

TESTS OF THYROID FUNCTION

1. **Measurement of circulating thyroid hormones**
   (i) Thyroxine (T_4)
       Affected by level of thyroid hormone-binding globulin (TBG)
       Does not detect T_3 thyrotoxicosis (e.g in iodine deficiency)
   (ii) Tri-iodothyronine (T_3)
       Detects T_3 thyrotoxicosis
   (iii) T_3 resin-uptake
       Determined by the degree of saturation of TBG with thyroid hormone
   (iv) Protein-bound iodine (PBI)
   (v) 'Free thyroxine index'
       The product of PBI and T_3 resin uptake. It is independent of the level of TBG
   (vi) Thyrotrophin (TSH)
       Increased in primary but not secondary hypothyroidism

(*contd*)

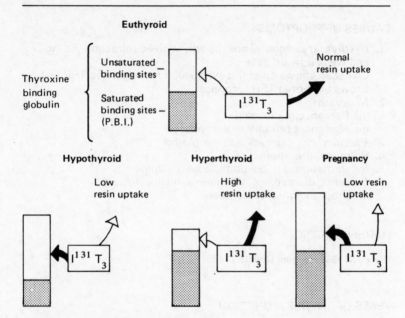

2. TRH test

The TSH response following intra-venous TRH is now replacing the T_3 suppression test for the diagnosis of thyroid autonomy.

Hypothyroidism → an exaggerated rise of an already increased TSH.

Hyperthyroidism → no response of a depressed TSH. Useful for diagnosis of doubtful hyperthyroidism and ophthalmic Graves' disease

3. Peripheral tissue respose tests

Useful in diagnosis of hypothyroidism only
  (i)   Tendon reflex duration
  (ii) Se cholesterol
  (iii) ECG
  (iv) Clinical response to thyroxine

4. Radio-iodine uptake tests

Now rarely used

5. Perchlorate discharge test

Detects inability of thyroid to bind iodine (the commonest type of dyshormonogenesis)

FURTHER READING

Hoffenberg R 1981 Medicine International 1: 256
Havard C W H 1975 British Journal of Hospital Medicine 14: 239

THYROID HORMONE BINDING GLOBULIN (TBG)

Causes of increased TBG
1. Pregnancy, oestrogen therapy
2. Drugs, e.g. clofibrate, phenothiazines
3. Viral hepatitis
4. Myxoedema

Causes of decreased TBG
1. Hypoproteinaemia (e.g. nephrotic syndrome)
2. Acromegaly
3. Glucocorticoids, androgens and anabolic steroids
4. Malnutrition or major illness
5. Thyrotoxicosis

Causes of reduced TBG binding
1. Renal failure
2. Salicylates, phenytoin, phenylbutazone

FURTHER READING

Havard C W H 1975 British Journal of Hospital Medicine 14: 239
Hoffenberg R 1978 Medicine, 3rd series, 8: 392

HYPOTHALAMIC REGULATORY HORMONES

Thyrotrophin releasing hormone—TRH
Releases
    (i) TSH and prolactin in both sexes
   (ii) FSH in men
  (iii) GH in some patients with acromegaly and renal failure

Luteinising/Follicle-stimulating hormone releasing factor—LH/FSH-RH
Releases
    (i) LH and FSH in both sexes
   (ii) GH in some patients with acromegaly

Somatostatin—GH-RIH
Suppresses
    (i) GH in normal subjects and acromegalic patients
   (ii) TSH response to TRH
  (iii) TSH secretion in hypothyroidism
   (iv) ACTH secretion in Nelson's syndrome
           (post-adrenalectomy)
   (v) Insulin, glucagon and gastrin release

Conditions associated with an impaired TSH response to TRH
1. Thyroid disease
    (i) Hyperthyroidism
    (ii) Pre-hyperthyroidism
    (iii) Euthyroid patients being treated for hyperthyroidism
    (iv) Ophthalmic Graves' disease
    (v) Multinodular goitre
2. Hypothalamic disease
3. Acromegaly or hypopituitarism
4. Cushing's disease
5. Depression
6. Starvation
7. Drugs—glucocorticoids, thyroid hormones, L-dopa
8. Some normal people

FURTHER READING

Hall R, Gomez-Pan A In: Lant A F (ed) Advanced medicine, symposium II.
    Pitman, London, p 234

METABOLIC BONE DISEASE

Causes of osteomalacia and rickets
1. *Deficiency of cholecalciferol (vit. D)*
    (i) Prematurity, multiple pregnancy, prolonged breast feeding
        and lack of UV predispose to rickets
    (ii) Dietary
    (iii) Post-gastrectomy (probably dietary)
    (iv) Malabsorption (p. 50)
    (v) Anticonvulsants (liver enzyme induction)
2. *Renal causes*
    (i) Chronic renal failure
    (ii) Idiopathic hypercalciuria
    (iii) Fanconi syndrome (p. 164)
    (iv) Tubular acidosis
3. *Hepatic disease (disturbed vit. D metabolism)*
4. *Hypo-phosphatasia*

Causes of osteoporosis
1. Senile osteoporosis
2. Immobilisation
3. Endocrine
    Sex hormone deficiency, e.g. premature menopause
    Cushing's or glucocorticoid therapy
    Hyperthyroidism
    Diabetes mellitus

4. Deficiency of oestrogen, androgen, protein, vit. C or calcium
5. Chronic renal failure
6. Miscellaneous
   Alcoholism
   Osteogenesis imperfecta
   Werner Rothmund syndrome
   Glycogen storage disease
   Cirrhosis in children
   Systemic mastocytosis or heparin infusion
   Homocystinuria
7. Localized osteoporosis, e.g. rheumatoid arthritis
8. Idiopathic osteoporosis of young people

FURTHER READING

Nordin C 1978 Medicine, 3rd series 10: 491

Types of hepatic osteodystrophy
1. Osteomalacia (mainly due to lack of vitamin D substrate)
2. Osteoporosis
3. Periosteal reaction with new bone formation
4. Secondary hyperparathyroidism (very rare)

FURTHER READING

Long R G, Wills M R 1978 British Journal of Hospital Medicine 20: 312

Causes of hypocalcaemia
1. Hypoparathyroidism
   (i) Post-thyroidectomy
   (ii) Idiopathic (sometimes with hypoadrenalism and
        Candidosis)
2. Deficiency of cholecalciferol (p. 150)
3. Malabsorption
4. Chronic renal failure or Fanconi syndrome (p. 164)
5. Hypoalbuminaemia
6. Neonatal hypocalcaemia
   (i) High-phosphate artificial feeds
   (ii) Associated with low birth-weight and hypoglycaemia
   (iii) Parathyroid suppression due to maternal
        hyperparathyroidism
7. Acute pancreatitis
8. Pseudo-hypoparathyroidism

	Response to parathormone infusion	Plasma PTH level
Idiopathic hypoparathyroidism	Urinary cAMP increases	Low
Pseudo-hypoparathyroidism	No response	Elevated

Causes of hypercalcaemia
1. Hyperparathyroidism
2. Malignancy with or without metastases
3. Myelomatosis, (rarely lymphoma or leukaemia)
4. Vit. D sensitivity, especially sarcoidosis
5. Vit. D excess
6. Milk-alkali syndrome
7. Infantile hypercalcaemia
8. Thyrotoxicosis
9. Hypothyroidism, especially in infants
10. Acute renal failure in polyuric phase
11. Steroid withdrawal (iatrogenic, or acute hypoadrenalism)
12. Paget's disease (when immobilised)
13. Immobilisation (very rarely)

FURTHER READING

Bailey J D et al 1978 Medicine, 3rd series, 10: 474
Martin J T, Larkins R G 1981 Medicine International 1: 267

Causes of hypercalciuria
1. All causes of hypercalcaemia, if renal function is normal
2. Renal tubular acidosis
3. Progressive osteoporosis
4. Cushing's syndrome
5. Acromegaly
6. Prolonged immobilisation
7. Excess dietary calcium
8. Idiopathic hypercalciuria

FURTHER READING

Smith L H, Williams H E 1971 In: Strauss M B, Welt L G (eds) Diseases of the kidney, 2nd edn. Little Brown, Boston, p 981

Tests to distinguish hyperparathyroidism from other causes of hypercalcaemia

1. *Steroid suppression test*
   Hypercalcaemia due to hyperparathyroidism is not suppressed by cortisol 40 mg tds
2. *Plasma phosphate*
   Consistently low PO_4 suggests primary hyperparathyroidism
3. *Phosphate excretion tests* (e.g. PEI, p. 221)
   Based on blockage of net phosphate reabsorption by parathormone
4. *Acid-base status*
   Patients with hyperparathyroidism have hyperchloraemic acidosis
   Other hypercalcaemic patients have hypochloraemic alkalosis
5. *Parathormone radioimmunoassay*
6. *Plasma alkaline phosphatase*
   Increased in patients with X-ray signs of hyperparathyroidism (osteoblastic activity)
7. *Calcium tolerance tests* (urinary phosphate excretion after calcium infusion)
   Parathormone production is not suppressed in hyperparathyroidism. Of limited value due to false positives and negatives

FURTHER READING

Martin J T, Larkins R G 1981 Medicine International 1: 267

Causes of soft-tissue calcification

1. *Dystrophic*
   Occurs in abnormal tissue, often with impaired blood supply.
   (i) Inflammatory foci, e.g. TB
   (ii) Neoplasia and naevi
   (iii) Parasites, e.g. cysticercosis
   (iv) Haematoma
   (v) Gravitational oedema (esp. leg ulcers)
   (vi) Systemic sclerosis, dermatomyositis
   (vii) Ehlers-Danlos syndrome (cutis hyperelastica)
2. *Metastatic* (*metabolic*)
   Calcification of normal tissue, e.g. kidneys or arteries, due to a metabolic abnormality such as hypercalcaemia or hypervitaminosis D. Intra-cranial calcification occurs in hypoparathyroidism and pseudo-hypoparathyroidism
3. *Secondary to bone or joint disease*
   e.g. calcified cartilage, tendon or periosteum

(*contd*)

4. *Idiopathic calcification*
   (i) Calcinosis circumscripta
   (ii) Calcinosis universalis
   (iii) Myositis ossificans

FURTHER READING

Nordin B E C 1973 Metabolic bone and stone disease. Churchill Livingstone, Edinburgh, p 244

Causes of discrete translucencies in a skull X-ray
1. Hyperparathyroidism
2. Myelomatosis
3. Metastatic deposits, esp. neuroblastoma
4. Leukaemia
5. Sickle-cell anaemia
6. Histiocytosis X, esp. Hand-Schuller-Christian disease
7. Sarcoidosis
8. Congenital cranial lacunae

Causes of bilateral frontal 'bossing'
1. Paget's
2. Rickets
3. Achondroplasia
4. Congenital hydrocephalus
5. Basal cell naevi syndrome (Gorlin's)

Causes of 'bowing' of tibia
1. Paget's
2. Rickets
3. Syphilis or yaws
4. Polyostotic fibrous dysplasia (Albright's)

MULTIPLE ENDOCRINE ADENOMATOSIS SYNDROMES

Type I. Werner's syndrome
Tumours of parathyroid, pituitary and pancreas

Parathyroid Adenoma or hyperplasia in 90%

Pituitary Adenoma in 65% (usually nonfunctional)

Pancreas
- (i) Islet-cell tumours with peptic ulceration (Zollinger-Ellison)
- (ii) Insulinoma
- (iii) Glucagonoma, with necrolytic migratory erythema, stomatitis, weight loss and diabetes
- (iv) Delta-cell hyperplasia with watery diarrhoea, hypokolaemia and fasting achlorhydria (Werner-Morrison)

Other reported lesions include adrenal hyperplasia or tumour, various thyroid lesions, carcinoid, schwannoma and thymoma

Type II. Sipple's syndrome
Tumours of thyroid, adrenal medulla and occasionally parathyroid adenoma or hyperplasia

Thyroid Medullary carcinoma which may secrete calcitonin, ACTH, serotonin or prostaglandin

Adrenal Phaeochromocytoma ' which may be asymptomatic. Some patients also have the 'mucosal neuroma' syndrome with pigmentation, thick lips, tongue or eyelid neuromas, lax joints and a Marfanoid body habitus

FURTHER READING

Schimke R N 1976 Advances in Internal Medicine 21: 249

Conditions associated with familial phaeochromocytoma
1. Multiple endocrine adenomatosis, Type II
2. Neurofibromatosis (von Recklinghausen)
3. Cerebellar haemangioblastoma (von Hippel-Lindau)
4. Basal-cell naevi syndrome (Gorlin)

Renal disease

CAUSES OF CHRONIC RENAL FAILURE

1. *Glomerulonephritis*
   (i) Immune-complex nephritis
      Primary, e.g. post-Streptococcal
      Secondary, e.g. Henoch-Schönlein vasculitis
   (ii) Anti-glomerular basement membrane nephritis, e.g.
      Goodpasture's nephritis with pulmonary bleeding
2. *Infections*
   Chronic pyelonephritis
   Renal TB (now uncommon)
3. *Obstruction*
   Stone, stricture, stenosis, etc.
4. *Incomplete recovery from acute renal failure* (esp. cortical
   necrosis)
5. *Vascular*
   Ischaemia
   Hypertension
6. *'Collagen vasculilar' diseases*
   Systemic vasculitis (PN etc, p. 178)
   SLE
   Systemic sclerosis
   'Haemolytic uraemic' syndrome
   Thrombotic thrombocytopenia of Moschcowitz
7. *Metabolic*
   Diabetes mellitus
   Amyloidosis
   Gout
   Hypercalcaemia (p. 152)
   Chronic hypokalaemia
   Drugs (esp. analgesic abuse) and toxins (e.g. heavy metals)
   Dysproteinaemia (esp. myelomatosis)
8. *Primary tubular disease*
   Fanconi syndrome (p. 164)
   Tubular acidosis

9. *Congenital anomalies*
   Polycystic kidney
   Renal hypoplasia
10. *Miscellaneous rare diseases*
   e.g. Radiation nephritis
      Balkan nephropathy
      Angiokeratoma corporis diffusum (Fabry's disease)
      Alport's disese (familial nephritis with deafness)

FURTHER READING

Linton A 1979 Medicine, 3rd series, 25: 1285

DIALYSIS

Possible indications for short-term dialysis
1. Acute renal failure
   (i) Hyperkalaemia > 7 mmol/l
   (ii) Arterial pH < 7.15
   (iii) Blood urea > 35 mmol/l
   (iv) Rapidly rising blood urea
2. Fluid overload
3. Uncontrolled hypercalcaemia
4. Gross electrolyte disturbance
5. Poisoning with salicylates
                  barbiturates
                  ethanol
6. Acute-on-chronic renal failure prior to establishing conservative therapy

Possible indications for long-term haemodialysis
1. Failure of conservative management
2. Se. creatinine > 1200 μmols/l
3. GFR < 3 ml/min
4. Progression of bone disease
5. Progression of neuropathy
6. Onset of pericarditis (peritoneal dialysis may be necessary initially to avoid haemopericarditis)

Neurological complications of renal failure
1. Encephalopathy with dementia
2. Epilepsy
3. Psychoses, esp. depression
4. Amaurosis
5. Cerebro-vascular accident
6. Basal ganglia lesions (tremor, rigidity, etc.)

7. Cranial neuropathy
8. Central pontine myelopathy
9. Peripheral neuropathy
10. Myopathy or muscle cramps
11. 'Restless leg' syndrome
12. Complications of therapy, e.g. viral or fungal CNS infection due to immunosuppressives
13. Lymphoma of CNS following renal transplant

FURTHER READING

Neary D 1976 British Journal of Hospital Medicine 15: 122

Renal causes of polycythaemia
1. Hypernephroma
2. Polycystic disease
3. Hydronephrosis
4. Renal artery stenosis
5. Transplantation

GLOMERULONEPHRITIS

Histological classification
1. *Minimal lesion* (no change on light microscopy)
2. *Membranous* (no cellular proliferation)
3. *Proliferative glomerulonephritis (PGN)*
   Each of the 3 cellular elements, epithelial, endothelial or mesangial, may show proliferative changes together or singly.
   (i) Active diffuse endothelial PGN
   (ii) Mesangial PGN
   (iii) Rapidly progressive PGN with extensive epithelial crescents
   (iv) Mesangiocapillary PGN
   (v) Focal PGN (affects only some parts of some glomeruli)
   (vi) Chronic endothelial PGN
4. *Focal glomerulosclerosis*
5. *Advanced sclerosing lesions*

   3(i) and 3(ii) are commonly post-streptococcal

Clinical syndromes of glomerulonephritis
1. Acute nephritis
2. Nephrotic syndrome
3. Persistent proteinuria
4. Recurrent haematuria or loin pain
5. Chronic renal failure
6. Acute oliguric renal failure (rare)

Antigens implicated in glomerulonephritis
1. *Bacterial*
   Streptococcal (β haemolytic, type 12)
   Staphylococci (in bact. endocarditis and in 'shunt' nephritis)
   Mycobact. leprae
   Treponema pallidum
   Salmonella typhi
2. *Viral*
   Australia antigen, varicella, mumps, EB virus, Coxsackie B
3. *Protozoal*
   Plasmodium malariae, schistosoma, toxoplasma
4. *Others*
   DNA (in SLE)
   Thyroglobulin (in auto-immune thyroiditis)
   Cryoglobulin
   Tumour antigens
   Carcino-embryonic antigen (in Ca. colon)
   Drugs, e.g. penicillamine, heroin

FURTHER READING

Dunea G, Mamdani B H 1979 Medicine, 3rd series, 26: 1322
Sissons J G P 1975 Medicine, 2nd series, 6: 256

CAUSES OF NEPHROTIC SYNDROME

1. *Glomerulonephritis (p. 158)*
   Accounts for 80% of cases
2. *Metabolic*
   (i) Diabetes mellitus
   (ii) Amyloidosis
   (iii) Lymphoma
   (iv) Extra-renal malignancy, e.g. bronchus
        Dysproteinaemia, esp. myelomatosis
   (vi) Dermatoses
   (vii) Sickle cell anaemia
   (viii) Myxoedema
3. *'Collagen vascular' disease*
   esp. SLE and vasculitis
4. *Infection*
   (i) Malaria
   (ii) Cytomegalic inclusion disease
   (iii) Syphilis
   (iv) Bacterial endocarditis
   (v) Staphylococcal septicaemia
   (vi) Leprosy

(contd)

5. *Mechanical*
   Renal artery stenosis
   Renal vein thrombosis (may be cause or effect)
   Inf. vena caval thrombosis
   Constrictive pericarditis
   Renal carcinoma
   Chyluria
6. *Drugs*
   Mercurials, troxidone, penicillamine, gold etc.
7. *Hypersensitivity*
   (i) Se sickness, bee stings, poison ivy, pollen, etc.
   (ii) Smallpox vaccination
8. *Congenital and familial*

FURTHER READING

Mallick N 1979 Medicine, 3rd series, 26: 1316
Parfrey P S 1982 British Journal of Hospital Medicine 27: 155

Causes of renal vein thrombosis
1. Nephrotic syndrome of any cause
2. Renal amyloid
3. Hypernephroma
4. Trauma, including cannulation
5. Dehydration, especially in infancy

Causes of papillary necrosis
1. Analgesic abuse, esp. phenacetin
2. Obstructive uropathy, esp. with infection
3. Acute pyelonephritis, esp. in diabetes mellitus
4. Sickle cell disease
5. Renal TB
6. Dysproteinaemia

Chronic interstitial nephritis
Defined as renal disease with the histological features of chronic pyelonephritis but with no evidence of bacterial infection. Many renal diseases produce interstitial changes, including:
1. Obstruction
2. Nephrocalcinosis
3. Potassium depletion
4. Hyperuricaemia
5. Analgesic abuse
6. Acute tubular necrosis
7. Irradiation
8. Lead poisoning
9. Balkan nephropathy

FURTHER READING

Freedman L R 1971 In: Strauss M B, Welt L G (eds) Diseases of the kidney, 2nd edn. Little Brown, Boston, p 667

Causes of 'sterile' pyuria
1. Renal TB
2. Analgesic nephropathy
3. Renal calculi
4. Urinary infection treated with chemotherapy
5. Drugs
   (i) Analgesics
   (ii) Diuretics
   (iii) Iron sorbitol citric acid complex (Jectofer)
6. Non-specific urethritis

NEPHROCALCINOSIS AND RENAL STONES

Causes of renal stones
1. *Calcium stones* (oxalate, phosphate, mixed magnesium-ammonium, etc.)
   (i) With hypercalcaemia
       Primary hyperparathyroidism
       Sarcoidosis
       Idiopathic hypercalcaemia of infancy
       Chronic milk-alkali syndrome
       Vit. D excess
   (ii) With normocalcaemia
       Idiopathic hypercalciuria
       Prolonged bed rest
       Primary renal tubular acidosis
       Urinary tract infection
       Hyperoxaluria
       Medullary sponge kidney
2. *Uric acid stones*
   (i) With hyperuricaemia
       Gout
       Polycythaemia, leukaemia, malignancy, etc.
       Chronic metabolic acidosis, e.g. glycogen storage disease
       Lesch-Nyhan syndrome
   (ii) With normouricaemia
       Idiopathic
       Acid, concentrated urine (e.g. desert climates)

(contd)

3. *Cystine stones*
   (i) Congenital cystinuria
   (ii) Hereditary cystinosis

Radio-opaque stones	Non-opaque stones
Calcium	Uric acid
Mg-ammonium phosphate	Xanthine
Cystine	Matrix
Silicate	

Differential diagnosis
   Blood clot
   Sloughed papillae
   Tumour
   Varices

Radiographic nephrocalcinosis
1. *Coarse, medullary*

Causes
   (i) Primary
       hyperparathyroidism
   (ii) Primary renal tubular
        acidosis
   (iii) Sarcoidosis
   (iv) Milk-alkali syndrome
   (v) Primary hyperoxaluria
       (oxalosis)
   (vi) Idiopathic hypercalciuria
   (vii) Idiopathic

2. *Localised*

Causes
   (i) Medullary sponge kidney
       (calcified collecting ducts)
   (ii) Renal neoplasm
   (iii) Cyst or haematoma
   (iv) Papillary necrosis
   (v) TB
   (vi) Hydatid cyst

3. *Diffuse, cortical(Rare)*

Causes
   (i) Chronic glomerulonephritis
   (ii) Old cortical necrosis

FURTHER READING

Wrong O M, Feest T G 1976 In: Peters D K (ed) Advanced medicine, symposium 12. Pitman, London, p 394

Execretion urography in acute renal failure
Now regarded as safe, providing dehydration is avoided (especial care needed in patients with liver failure, diabetes and myelomatosis)
The evolution of the nephrogram is helpful:

Type 1. Immediate, faint, persisting
   Chronic glomerulo-nephritis

Type 2. Increasingly dense with time
   Obstruction
   Hypotension or ischaemia
   Severe glomerulonephritis

Type 3. Immediate, dense, persisting
   Acute tubular necrosis
   Oliguric pyelonephritis

Type 4. No nephrogram
   Anuric glomerulonephritis
   Renal infarction
   Severe interstitial nephritis
In obstructive uropathy there may also be asymmetry of renal size, and a slowly developing dense pyelogram

FURTHER READING

Cattell W R 1975 In: Jones N F (ed) Recent advances in renal disease—1. Churchill Livingstone, Edinburgh, p 21
Fry I K 1975 Medicine, 2nd series, 29: 1618

Causes of small kidneys
   1. Chronic glomerulonephritis (smooth outline)
   2. Chronic pyelonephritis (irregular outline)
   3. Other chronic nephropathy, e.g. interstitial nephritis
   4. Renal artery stenosis
   5. Atrophy following obstruction
   6. Congenital renal hypoplasia (prone to infection)

Causes of large kidney (or kidneys)
1. Polycystic disease or solitary cyst
2. Hydronephrosis or pyonephrosis
3. Hypernephroma
4. Hypertrophy following contra-lateral nephrectomy or failure
5. Nephrotic syndrome
6. Acute pyelonephritis
7. Compulsive water, beer or cider drinker

Also consider the possibility of peri-renal haematoma

RENAL TUBULAR DISORDERS

Single transport defects
1. *Impaired reabsorption*
   Water—nephrogenic diabetes insipidus
   Na or K—distal tubular damage, e.g. chronic pyelonephritis
   Calcium—idiopathic hypercalciuria
   Phosphate—vitamin D resistant rickets
   Glucose—renal glycosuria
   Amino acids—see page 165
   Xanthine—xanthinuria
2. *Excessive reabsorption*
   Phosphate—pseudo-hypoparathyroidism

Multiple transport defects
1. *Impaired acidification*
    (i) Renal tubular acidosis
   (ii) Chronic pyelonephritis
   (iii) Hypokalaemia
   (iv) Hypercalcaemia
   (v) Hydronephrosis
2. *Impaired reabsorption and acidification*
   (Fanconi syndrome) e.g.
    (i) Hereditary cystinosis (Lignac-Fanconi)
   (ii) Toxins—cadmium, Hg, lead
   (iii) Drugs—neomycin, outdated tetracycline
   (iv) Galactosaemia
   (v) Hepatolenticular degeneration
   (vi) Nephrotic syndrome
   (vii) Lowe's oculo-cerebro-renal syndrome

FURTHER READING

Gabriel R 1974 Postgraduate nephrology. Butterworth, London, p 142

AMINO-ACIDURIA

Four groups with separate transport systems
1. Proline, hydroxyproline and glycine
2. Dibasic: cystine, ornithine, arginine and lysine (COAL)
3. Dicarboxylic: glutamic and aspartic acids
4. Monoamino-monocarboxylic: all the rest

Causes of aminoaciduria
1. *Pure 'overflow'* due to raised plasma levels
   Amino-acid infusion
   Liver failure
   Phenylketonuria
   Maple-syrup urine
   Histidinaemia
   Glycinaemia
2. *A specific transport defect*
   Cystinuria
   Hartnup disease (malabsorption, ataxia and pellagrous rash)
3. *Generalised proximal tubular damage* (Fanconi syndrome)
4. *Mixed 'overflow' and renal*
   Citrullinuria
   Prolinaemia

SOME CAUSES OF 'DARK COLOURED' URINE

1. Concentration
2. Bile
3. Blood, haemoglobinuria or myoglobinuria
4. Methaemoglobinuria
5. Porphyria
6. Alkaptonuria
7. Melaninuria
8. Beetroot, dyes in sweets, etc.

DRUG-INDUCED RENAL DISEASE

1. **Acute renal failure** (20% of cases are due to drugs)
   Over 70 drugs implicated, and a variety of mechanisms,
   (i) Direct toxicity (dose-related)
       e.g. cephaloridine, amphotericin B
   (ii) Hypersensitivity
       e.g. penicillin, sulphonamides
   (iii) Obstruction due to crystal formation
       e.g. sulphonamides
   (iv) 'Osmotic nephrosis'
       e.g. low MW dextran infusion

(contd)

Tetracyclines cause two distinct disorders:
  a. Renal failure (due to increased urea production, increased sodium excretion and reduced urine-concentrating ability)
  b. Degraded tetracyclines cause proximal tubular defects (Fanconi syndrome)
2. **Drug-induced LE**
  (especially in slow acetylators)
3. **Nephrotic syndrome** (p. 159)
4. **Papillary necrosis**
  Analgesics, especially phenacetin
5. **Retro-peritoneal fibrosis**
  e.g. methysergide, ergotamine, methyldopa
6. **Metabolic effects**
   (i) Increased protein breakdown, e.g. glucocorticoids
   (ii) Electrolyte disturbance, e.g. drugs causing diarrhoea
   (iii) Nephrocalcinosis, e.g. vitamin D overdosage
   (iv) Renal calculi, e.g. 'milk-alkali' syndrome
   (v) Urate nephropathy, e.g. cytotoxins for malignancy
   (vi) Impaired urine-concentrating ability, e.g. demethylchlortetracycline, lithium
   (vii) Inappropriate ADH secretion (p. 171)
7. **Neoplasm**
  Renal pelvis mesothelial tumour, e.g. analgesics

FURTHER READING

Curtis J R 1977 British Medical Journal 2: 242, 375.
Curtis J R 1980 British Journal of Hospital Medicine 24: 29

ACID-BASE BALANCE

These headings reflect changes in extra-cellular fluid only, e.g. in metabolic alkalosis there is an associated intra-cellular acidosis

1. RESPIRATORY ACIDOSIS (Low pH, High CO_2 content)
   Any cause of hypoventilation (p. 27)
2. RESPIRATORY ALKALOSIS (High pH, Low CO_2 content)
   Any cause of hyperventilation (p. 27)
3. METABOLIC ACIDOSIS (Low pH, Low CO_2 content)
   Causes
   (i) Ingestion of hydrion or 'potential acid'
       Diets high in protein and fat
           Ammonium chloride, salicylates, calcium chloride, etc.
           'Dilution acidaemia' due to rapid saline infusion
   (ii) *Metabolic overproduction of hydrions*
        Hypercatabolic states
        Ketosis, e.g. starvation, diabetes mellitus
        Lactic acidosis (p. 168)
   (iii) *Intestinal loss of base*
         Diarrhoea
         Fistulae
   (iv) *Renal causes*
        a. Acute or chronic failure
        b. Defective hydrion secretion
           Renal tubular acidosis
           Pyelonephritis
           Hydronephrosis
        c. Extra-renal causes
               Carbonic anhydrase inhibitors
               Addison's disease
               Uretero-sigmoidostomy
4. METABOLIC ALKALOSIS (High pH, High CO_2 content)
   Causes
   Ingestion of alkali, e.g. $NaHCO_3$
   Vomiting, or gastric aspiration
   Hypokalaemia (p. 168)
5. MIXED DISORDERS
   e.g. Respiratory and meatabolic acidosis in hypoventilated
        hypoxic patients
        Respiratory alkalosis and metabolic acidosis in salicylate
        poisoning

FURTHER READING

Flenley D C 1978 British Journal of Hospital Medicine 20: 384
Gardner M L G 1978 Medical aid-base balance, Bailliere Tindall, London

Causes of lactic acidosis
1. *Poor tissue perfusion or hypoxia,* e.g. 'shock'
2. *Metabolic disease*
   Renal failure
   Hepatic failure
   Infection
   Diabetes mellitus
3. *Drugs*
   Phenformin or metformin
   Ethanol or methanol
   Fructose, etc.
4. *Ingestion of 'lactic acid' milk*
5. *Congenital*
   G6P deficiency, etc.

N.B. An increased anion gap $([Na^+] + [K^+]) - ([Cl^-] + [HCO_3^-])$ is helpful in diagnosis if blood lactate estimation cannot be performed.

FURTHER READING

Alberti K G M M, Natress M 1977 Lancet 2: 25
Cohen R D 1980 British Journal of Hospital Medicine 24: 577

Causes of hypokalaemia
1. *Increased renal loss*
   (i) Diuresis
       Drugs
       Diabetes mellitus
   (ii) Minerolocorticoid excess
       Primary aldosteronism (Conn's tumour)
       Cushing's
       Ingestion of liquorice or carbenexolone
   (iii) Primary renal disease
       Diuretic phase of acute renal failure
       Chronic pyelonephritis
       Fanconi syndrome (p. 164)
       Renal tubular acidosis
       Renal ischaemia

2. *Increased intestinal loss*
   Diarrhoea
   Vomiting
   Aspiration
   Fistulae
   Resonium A
3. *Decreased intake*
   Dietary lack
   Malabsorption
4. *Familial periodic paralysis*
5. *I.V. insulin*

FURTHER READING

Wilkinson R 1975 Medicine, 2nd series, 7: 334

Causes of hypernatraemia
1. *Inadequate water intake*
   Lack of water, inability to drink, etc.
2. *Inadequate water retention*
   Diabetes insipidus
3. *Excessive sodium intake*
   Diet or drugs (oral or intravenous)
4. *Excessive sodium retention*
   Hyperaldosteronism

Causes of hyponatraemia
1. *Excessive water intake*
   Oral (polydipsia) or intravenous
2. *Excessive water retention*
   Inappropriate ADH secretion
3. *Inadequate sodium intake* (rare)
4. *Inadequate sodium retention*
   (i) Vomiting, diarrhoea
   (ii) Hypoadrenalism
   (iii) 'Salt-losing nephritis'

FURTHER READING

Davison A M 1980 Medicine, 3rd series, 26: 1356
Thompson F D 1979 British Journal of Hospital Medicine 21: 46
Sanderson P 1978 Medicine, 3rd series, 11: 565

Drugs causing sodium and water retention

1. Corticosteroids and corticotrophin, e.g. fludrocortisone
2. Oestrogens
3. Anti-inflammatory drugs, e.g. phenylbutazone
4. Carbenoxolone and liquorice-like compounds
5. Vasodilators, e.g. minoxidil, diazoxide
6. Hypotensives (esp. at start of therapy) e.g. guanethidine
7. Psychotropic drugs, e.g. lithium
8. Sodium-containing drugs, e.g. liquid antacids
         carbenecillin
         X-ray contrast media

FURTHER READING

Brown Edwina A, MacGregor G A 1981 Prescribers' Journal 21: 251

CAUSES OF JAUNDICE WITH URAEMIA

1. Infections
 (i) Gram-negative septicaemia
 (ii) Leptospirosis icterohaemorrhagiae (Weil's)
 (iii) Yellow fever
2. Drugs and toxins
 (i) Direct toxicity e.g. carbon tetrachloride
 (ii) Hypersensitivity e.g. penicillin
3. Hepatorenal syndrome
 Oliguria secondary to hepatic failure, usually following
 biliary tract surgery or cirrhosis
4. Haemolytic-uraemic syndrome
5. Incompatible blood transfusion
6. Toxaemia of pregnancy
7. Other causes of 'shock'

FURTHER READING

Wilkinson S P 1975 Medicine, 2nd series, 29: 1647

CAUSES OF POLYDIPSIA AND POLYURIA

1. *Decreased vasopressin production*
 (i) Cranial diabetes insipidus
  Congenital
  Head injury or neurosurgery
  Tumours e.g. craniopharyngioma
  Sarcoid, histiocytosis X, TB, etc.
 (ii) Psychogenic polydipsia

2. *Decreased renal tubular response to vasopressin*
   (i) Congenital nephrogenic diabetes insipidus
   (ii) Hypercalcaemia or hypokalaemia
   (iii) Chronic renal failure
   (iv) Obstructive uropathy
   (v) Lithium therapy, demeclocycline
   (vi) Psychogenic polydipsia
3. *Osmotic diuresis*
   (i) Heavy glycosuria
   (ii) Mannitol therapy
4. *Dry mouth*
   Sjögren's syndrome

FURTHER READING

Baylis P H 1981 Medicine International 1: 249
Edwards C P W 1975 In: Lant A F (ed) Advanced medicine, symposiumm II.
  Pitman, London, p 276

ARGININE VASOPRESSIN (Antidiuretic hormone)

Causes of inappropriate ADH secretion
1. *Neoplasm*
   Ectopic synthesis, especially bronchial oat-cell Ca.
2. *Neuro-hypophyseal disease*
   Intra-cranial inflammation, bleeding, tumour, trauma, etc.
3. *Non-neoplastic thoracic disease*
   TB, pneumonia, cardiac surgery
4. *Endocrine*
   Hypoadrenalism, hypothyroidism, hypopituitarism
5. *Drugs*
   Chlorpropamide
   Carbamazepine
   Cyclophosphamide
   Clofibrate
   Thiazides
6. *Miscellaneous*
   Pain, trauma, hypotension, leukaemia, lymphoma

FURTHER READING

Baylis P H 1981 Medicine International 1: 249
Thompson F D 1979 British Journal of Hospital Medicine 21: 46

Rheumatology

RAYNAUD'S PHENOMENON

Paroxysmal digital ischaemia, usually accompanied by pallor and cyanosis and followed by erythema

Causes
1. *Reflex vasoconstriction*
   (i) Raynaud's disease
   (ii) Cervical spondylosis
   (iii) Shoulder-hand syndrome
   (iv) Vibrating machinery
2. *Arterial occlusion*
   (i) Thoracic outlet syndromes (p. 180)
   (ii) Embolus, thrombosis or stenosis
   (iii) Arteriosclerosis
   (iv) Buerger's disease
   (v) Injury (Volkmann's ischaemia)
3. *'Collagen vascular' disease*
   (i) Systemic sclerosis
   (ii) Polyarteritis
   (iii) SLE
   (iv) Rh. arthritis, Sjøgren's
4. *Increased blood agglutination*
   (i) Cold agglutinins
   (ii) Dysproteinaemias
   (iii) Polycythaemia, leukaemia, Moschcowitz's, etc.
5. *Neurological:* paralysis or disuse of a limb
6. *Cold injury:* frost bite
7. *Toxins*
   (i) Vinyl chloride
   (ii) Ergot
   (iii) Heavy metals
   (iv) Tobacco
8. *Drugs:* β-blockers
9. *Malnutrition and cachexia*
10. *Miscellaneous rare causes*
    Typhoid fever, amyloidosis, myxoedema etc.

FURTHER READING

Birnstingl M 1979 British Journal of Hospital Medicine 21: 602

Causes of cryoglobulinaemia
1. Idiopathic
2. Collagen-vascular disease
3. Infections
    Bacterial endocarditis
    Syphilis
    Infectious mononucleosis
    Cytomegalic virus infection
    Leprosy
    Kala-azar
    Toxoplasmosis
4. Multiple myeloma and Waldenstrøm's macroglobulinaemia
5. Myeloproliferative disease
6. Miscellaneous
    Sickle-cell disease
    Glomerulonephritis
    Myocardial infarction
    Ulcerative colitis
    Chronic liver disease, etc.

RHEUMATOID DISEASE

ARA criteria for diagnosis of rheumatoid arthritis
1. Morning stiffness
2. Pain and tenderness in at least one joint
3. Swelling of one joint for six weeks or more
4. Swelling in another joint
5. Symmetrical joint swelling
6. Subcutaneous nodules
7. Periarticular osteoporosis, bony erosions
8. Positive test for rheumatoid factor
9. Poor mucin precipitate of synovial fluid
10. Typical synovial histology
11. Typical nodule histology

Classical rheumatoid = 7 of above
Definite rheumatoid = 5 of above
Probable rheumatoid = 3 of above

FURTHER READING

Bluestone R, Bacon P A 1977 Clinics in Rheumatic Diseases 3, No 3,
    Saunders, Philadelphia
Katz W A 1977 Rheumatic diseases, diagnosis and management. Lippincott,
    Philadelphia, p 421

Complications of rheumatoid disease

1. *Poor general health*
    (i) Weight loss
    (ii) Anaemia
    (iii) Depression and social problems
2. *Joint complications*
    (i) Deformity, subluxation, etc.
    (ii) Pyoarthrosis
    (iii) Tendon rupture, due to attrition or nodules
    (iv) Nerve compression due to tenosynovial swelling
    (v) Cord or root compression, due to cervical subluxation
    (vi) Baker's synovial cyst
    (vii) Acute rupture of synovial sac, especially in knee
    (viii) Hoarseness, due to crico-arytenoid arthritis
    (ix) Deafness, due to arthritis of auditory ossicles
3. *Pressure sores and infected ulcers*
4. *Osteoporosis and muscle atrophy*
5. *Pulmonary*
    (i) Pleuritis, effusion
    (ii) Nodule in lung or pleura
    (iii) Fibrosing alveolitis
    (iv) Caplan's syndrome in pneumoconiosis
6. *Cardiac*
    (i) Pericarditis
    (ii) Rheumatoid granuloma of heart
7. *Ocular*
    (i) Scleritis
    (ii) Scleromalacia perforans
    (iii) Sjøgren's syndrome
8. *Arteritis*
    (i) Digital ischaemia (may be Raynaud's)
    (ii) Leg ulcers
    (iii) Mesenteric ischaemia
    (iv) Arteritis of lungs, kidneys, liver, etc.
9. *Peripheral and autonomic neuropathy*
10. *Lymphadenopathy*
    Usually in region of an inflamed joint
11. *Amyloidosis*
    May develop renal vein thrombosis
12. Hyperviscosity syndrome due to macromolecule polymerization (esp. R A factor)
13. *Felty's syndrome* (Splenomegaly, RA and leucopenia)
14. *Complications of therapy*
15. *Associated auto-immune disease*
    (i) Pernicious anaemia
    (ii) Thyroiditis
    (iii) Haemolytic anaemia, etc.
16. *Subfertility* (Prior to development of arthritis)

FURTHER READING

Holland C, Jayson M I V 1978 Medicine, 3rd series, 12: 575
Hughes G R V 1979 British Journal of Hospital Medicine 21: 584

Factors in the anaemia of RA
1. Fe deficiency
    (i) GI blood loss due to drugs (aspirin, indomethacin, butazolidine, glucocorticoids)
    (ii) Defective Fe utilization ('anaemia of chronic disorders')
2. Folic acid deficiency
3. Marrow hypoplasia
4. Haemodilution
5. Haemolysis, especially in Felty's syndrome
6. Increased incidence of pernicious anaemia

Conditions in which rheumatoid factor may be present
1. Collagen vascular disease, especially Sjøgren's syndrome and rheumatoid disease
2. Infection
    (i) Syphilis
    (ii) Kala-azar
    (iii) Leprosy
    (iv) Infective endocarditis
    (v) Tuberculosis
    (vi) Rubella
    (vii) Infectious mononucleosis
3. Sarcoidosis
4. Asbestosis
5. Chronic liver disease
6. Post-blood transfusion
7. Malignancy
8. Waldenstrøm's macroglobulinaemia
9. Renal transplantation
10. Glomerulonephritis
11. Relatives of RA patients
12. Normal old age

FURTHER READING

Mowat A G 1978 Medicine, 3rd series, 12: 590

Conditions associated with Sjøgren's syndrome
1. Collagen-vascular disease
2. Hashimoto's thyroiditis
3. Peripheral neuropathy
4. Renal tubular acidosis
5. Primary biliary cirrhosis
6. Diffuse interstitial pulmonary fibrosis
7. Cryoglobulinaemia
8. Hyperglobulinaemic purpura (Waldenstrøm)
9. Lymphoma
10. Pancreatitis

LUPUS ERYTHEMATOSUS

ARA Criteria for diagnosis of SLE
1. Facial erythema
2. Discoid lupus
3. Raynaud's phenomenon
4. Alopecia
5. Photosensitivity
6. Oral or nasopharyngeal ulceration
7. Arthritis without deformity
8. LE cells
9. Chronic false positive WR
10. Profuse proteinuria
11. Cellular casts
12. Pleurisy or pericarditis
13. Haemolytic anaemia, leukopenia or thrombocytopenia
14. Psychosis or convulsions

The presence of four or more features strongly suggests SLE

FURTHER READING

Bresnihan B 1979 British Journal of Hospital Medicine 22: 16
Cohen A S et al 1971 Bulletin of Rheumatic Diseases 21: 643

Conditions in which antinuclear antibodies may be present
1. Collagen vascular disease, esp. SLE
2. Chronic liver disease
3. Hashimoto's thyroiditis, thymoma, myasthenia gravis
4. Pernicious anaemia
5. Tuberculosis
6. Leprosy
7. Diffuse pulmonary fibrosis
8. Lymphoma or other malignancy
9. Ulcerative colitis
10. Normal old people

FURTHER READING

Holborow E J 1978 British Journal of Hospital Medicine 19: 250

Patterns of nuclear fluorescence

Pattern	Antigen	Found in:
Diffuse	DNA	SLE, rheumatoid and other collagen-vascular disease
Peripheral (*'shaggy'*)	DNA	Active SLE with nephritis or vasculitis
Nucleolar	RNA	Mainly systemic sclerosis
Speckled	(i) SM RNA-ase resistant	Mainly SLE
	(ii) Extractable nuclear antigen RNA-ase sensitive	Mixed connective tissue disease

FURTHER READING

Biundo J J, Cummings N A 1977 In: Katz W A (ed) Rheumatic diseases, diagnosis and management, Lippincott, Philadelphia, p 269
Holborow E J 1978 British Journal of Hospital Medicine 19: 250

NECROTIZING VASCULITIS

No classification is completely satisfactory, since the clinical syndromes may overlap, and their pathogenesis is imperfectly understood.

1. *Polyarteritis nodosa*
   (i) Classical systemic
   (ii) Cutaneous
2. *Giant cell arteritis*
   i) Cranial arteritis
   (ii) Polymyalgia rheumatica
   (iii) Aortic arch syndrome (including Takayasu's)
3. *Granulomatous*
   (i) Wegener's granuloma and lethal midline granuloma
   (ii) Allergic granulomatosis (Churg)
   (iii) Lymphomatoid granulomatosis
4. *Rheumatic and collagen diseases*
   (i) Rheumatoid
   (ii) SLE
   (iii) Dermatomyositis
   (iv) Systemic sclerosis
   (v) Rheumatic fever
5. *Leukocytoclastic* (neutrophilic infiltrate with nuclear fragmentation).
   (i) Leukocytoclastic vasculitis (Zeek)
   (ii) Henoch-Schönlein purpura
   (iii) Hypocomplementaemic vasculitis (often urticarial)
   (iv) Essential mixed cryoglobulinaemia
   (v) Hyperglobulinaemic purpura (Waldenström)
   (vi) Erythema nodosum, nodular vasculitis or erythema induration
   (vii) Erythema elevatum diutinum
6. *Infective*
   (i) Extension of perivascular inflammation, e.g. cellulitis, abscess
   (ii) Septicaemia, septic emboli
   (iii) Cutaneous arteritis during rash of meningococcaemia, scarlatina, typhus fever etc.

FURTHER READING

Sams W M Jr 1980 Journal of the American Academy of Dermatology 3: 1
Travers R L 1979 Britain Journal of Hospital Medicine 22: 38

Causes of hypermobile joints
1. Marfan's
2. Ehlers-Danlos
3. Osteogenesis imperfecta
4. Inflammatory polyarthritis, e.g. RA
5. Charcot's arthropathy
6. Homocystinuria
7. Hyperlysinaemia
8. Idiopathic

Causes of generalised stiffness
1. *Unaccustomed exercise*
2. *Systemic infection, e.g. influenza*
3. *Arthritis*, especially
    (i) Rheumatoid
    (ii) Polymyalgia rheumatica
    (iii) Generalised osteoarthrosis
    (iv) Ochronosis
    (v) Haemochromatosis
    (vi) Serum sickness
4. *Neuromuscular disease*
    (i) 'Stiff man syndrome' (tonic muscle rigidity)
    (ii) Cervical spondylosis with myelopathy
    (iii) Extrapyramidal disease
        Torsion dystonia
        Hepato-lenticular degeneration (Wilson's)
        Parkinsonism
    (iv) Tetanus
    (v) McArdle's myopathy
    (vi) Myotonia
    (vii) Dermatomyositis
5. *Scleroderma* (p. 187)
6. *Generalised oedema*
    (i) Anascara
    (ii) Scleroedema
    (iii) Erythroderma
7. *Hypothyroidism*, especially in cold weather
8. *Mucopolysaccharidoses* (p. 184)

The 'shoulder-hand syndrome' (Sudek's atrophy)

Associated conditions
1. Myocardial infarction
2. Trauma
3. Cervical spinal lesion
4. Hemiplegia
5. Brain tumour
6. Epilepsy (? phenobarbitone)

(contd)

7. Electro-convulsive therapy
8. Pulmonary lesions
9. Herpes zoster
10. Panniculitis
11. Vasculitis

Causes of carpal tunnel syndrome
1. Idiopathic
2. Pregnancy, 'Pill', pre-menstrual
3. Myxoedema
4. Acromegaly
5. Rheumatoid arthritis (may be presenting symptom)
6. Previous scaphoid fracture
7. Intermittent trauma
8. Mucopolysaccharidosis V (Scheie's syndrome)

FURTHER READING

Le Quesne P M 1977 British Journal of Hospital Medicine 17: 155

Thoracic outlet syndromes
1. Scalenus anticus
2. Cervical rib
3. Hyperabduction
4. Costoclavicular
5. Clavipectoral
6. Postural and sleep syndromes

Radiological features of some arthropathies

Osteo-arthrosis
1. New bone formation
     Osteophytes
     Peri-articular ossicles
     Loose bodies
2. Cartilage loss, often confined to weight-bearing surface
3. Sclerosis and subchondral cavitation
4. Juxta-articular cysts
5. Subluxation in advanced cases
6. **No** ankylosis

Ankylosing spondylitis
1. Bilateral erosive SI disease, with later sclerosis
2. Erosion in intervertebral facets and costo-vertebral joints
3. Calcified spinal ligaments
4. Erosion in limb joints, especially hips
5. Irregularity of weight-bearing surfaces
6. Calcification of the entheses

Rheumatoid arthritis
1. Juxta-articular osteoporosis
2. Cartilage loss
3. Marginal and surface erosions
4. Subluxations, dislocations and carpal ankylosis
5. **No** sclerosis or new bone formation

Chondrocalcinosis
Calcium deposits (punctate-linear opacities) are seen esp. in AP
view of knees, and in symphysis pubis and wrists.

Causes of a periosteal reaction
1. Osteomyelitis
2. Healing fracture
3. Rheumatoid arthritis (especially juvenile)
4. Hypertrophic pulmonary osteoarthropathy
5. Psoriatic arthritis
6. Reiter's syndrome
7. Cellulitis
8. Bone tumours, e.g. osteo-sarcoma
9. Subperiosteal haemorrhage, e.g. scurvy
10. Polyarteritis nodosa

Conditions associated with ankylosing spondylitis
1. Aortic insufficiency
2. Uveitis
3. Pulmonary fibrosis
4. Amyloidosis
5. Enteropathy—Ulcerative colitis
                              Crohn's disease
                              Whipple's disease
6. Psoriasis
7. Reiter's disease

CAUSES OF HYPERURICAEMIA

1. Increased purine synthesis
   (i) Primary gout (in 25% of cases)
   (ii) Lesch-Nyhan syndrome (Congenital mental deficiency, choreo-athetosis and lip chewing)

2. Increased turnover of preformed purines
   (i) Myeloproliferative disease and lymphoma
   (ii) Chronic haemolysis
   (iii) Psoriasis
   (iv) Fructose ingestion
   (v) High purine diet

3. Decreased renal excretion
   (i) Primary gout (in 75% of cases)
   (ii) Chronic renal failure
   (iii) Hyperparathyroidism
   (iv) Lead nephropathy
   (v) Down's syndrome
   (vi) Increased organic acid production:
   Exercise
   Starvation, vomiting
   Diabetic keto-acidosis
   Alcohol
   Toxaemia of pregnancy
   Glycogen storage disease (G6P deficiency)
   Hyperlipidaemia
   (vii) Drugs:
   Salicylates (in low dosage)
   Uricosurics (in low dosage)
   Diuretics
   Pyrazinamide
   Ethambutol

Se uric acid also tends to be high in patient with hypertension, obesity and high IQ

FURTHER READING

Nuki G 1975 In: Lant A F (ed) Advanced medicine, symposium II. Pitman, London, p 334

CALCIUM PYROPHOSPHATE ARTHROPATHY

Pseudogout (chondrocalcinosis) may mimic gout, rheumatoid arthritis, osteoarthrosis or neuropathic arthropathy
Numerous intraleucocytic crystals (CPPD) in synovial fluid are diagnostic

ASSOCIATED CONDITIONS

1. **Metabolic**
   Hyperuricaemia (with or without gout)
   Hyperparathyroidism
   Paget's disease of bone
   Hepato-lenticular degeneration (Wilson's)
   Haemochromatosis
   Acromegaly
   Ochronosis
   Hypophosphatasia
   Hypomagnesaemia
   Hypothyroidism
   Diabetes mellitus

2. **Hypertension or atheroma**
3. **Renal failure or calculi**
4. **Secondary to other arthropathies**
   Osteoarthrosis
   Neuropathic arthropathy
   Rheumatoid arthritis

5. **Idiopathic**

FURTHER READING

Yu T, Katz W A 1977 In: Katz W A (ed) Rheumatic diseases, diagnosis and management. Lippincott, Philadelphia, p 724
McCarty D J 1980 Advances in Internal Medicine, vol 25 Year Book Med. Pub. Inc, Chicago, p 363–390

INHERITED DISORDERS OF CONNECTIVE TISSUE

A. Defect in fibrous elements
1. *Primary disorder of biosynthesis of CT*
    (i) Ehlers-Danlos syndromes (at least 8 types)
    (ii) Osteogenesis imperfecta (deficiency of Type I collagen)
    (iii) Marfan syndrome (at least 4 types)
2. *Secondary damage to CT*
    (i) Alkaptonuria (defective homogentisic acid degradation)
    (ii) Homocystinuria (resembles the Marfan syndrome, but with thromboses and osteoporosis; due to a specific enzyme defect)
    (iii) Menkes 'kinky hair' syndrome (defective copper transport)
    (iv) Pseudo-xanthoma elasticum (degeneration of elastic fibres)

B. Mucopolysaccharidoses
Lysosomal storage diseases with disordered glycosaminoglycan degradation due to specific enzyme deficiencies

Type Clinical features	
I *Hurler*	Gargoylism, dwarfing, hepatosplenomegaly, mental deficiency, corneal opacity, deafness. Death in childhood.
II *Hunter*	A milder form, limited to males
III *Sanfilippo**	Severe CNS changes, minor somatic changes.
IV *Morquio*	Characteristic skeletal changes (dwarfing, knock-knee, barrel chest, etc), normal I.Q.
V *Scheie**	Stiff joints, coarse facies, corneal opacity.
VI *Maroteaux**	Similar to Hurler's but normal I.Q.
VII *Dygvve**	Similar to Morquio's but mentally retarded

*Very rare

FURTHER READING

McKusick V A 1976 In: Peters D K (ed) Advanced medicine, symposium 12. Pitman, London, p 170

Dermatology

SKIN CHANGES ASSOCIATED WITH SYSTEMIC MALIGNANCY

A. Genetic syndromes predisposing to neoplasm
1. Phakomatoses (Disseminated hamartomata of eye, skin and brain)
    - (i) Neurofibromatosis (von Recklinghausen's)
    - (ii) Epiloia (Bourneville's, tuberose sclerosis)
    - (iii) Basal cell naevoid syndrome (Gorlin's)
    - (iv) Cerebellar haemangioblastoma (von Hippel-Lindau)
    - (v) Encephalotrigeminal angiomatosis (Sturge-Weber's)
2. Familial tylosis (keratoderma) and Ca. oesophagus
3. Familiar polyposis coli (Gardner's) with sebaceous cysts
4. Defective immunosurveillance
    - (i) Wiskott-Aldrich
    - (ii) Ataxia telangiectasia
    - (iii) Chediak-Higashi
5. Small intestinal polyposis with perioral lentigines (Peutz-Jegher's syndrome). Rarely associated with carcinoma
6. Multiple endocrine adenomatosis (Type 2) with pigmentation, mucosal neuromas and medullary Ca. thyroid
7. Werner's premature ageing syndrome
8. Cowden's disease. Tricholemmomata on face, oral mucosa and hands antedating Ca. of breast, thyroid or female reproductive tract

B. Signs of exposure to a carcinogen
1. Nicotine staining of fingers
2. Signs of arsenic ingestion
    - (i) Keratoses
    - (ii) Diffuse pigmentation with 'rain-drops' of paler normal skin
3. Bowen's disease of covered skin
4. X-ray dermatitis or multiple basal cell ca. over spine may indicate increased risk of leukaemia

C. Direct involvement of skin by malignancy
1. Direct spread, e.g. carcinoma erysipeloides or carcinoma telangiectoides
2. Metastases
3. Paget's disease of skin (nipple or perineum)
4. Leukaemic infiltrate
5. Skin changes of lymphoma
    (i) Prelymphomatous poikiloderma
    (ii) Cutaneous spread of a systemic lymphoma
    (iii) Mycosis fungoides and Sezary's syndrome

D. Other associations
1. Pigmentation
2. Pallor
3. Pruritus (esp. lymphoma)
4. Acanthosis nigricans and papillomatosis (esp. GI malignancy)
5. Dermatomyositis
6. Hypertrophic pulmonary osteo-arthropathy (p. 41)
7. Herpes zoster (esp. lymphoma)
8. Acquired ichthyosis (esp. lymphoma)
9. Figurate erythema, e.g. Erythema gyratum repens
10. Rapid onset of multiple basal-cell papillomata (Leser-Trelat)
11. Hypertrichosis lanuginosa (acquired)
12. Widespread viral infection (eczema herpeticum, etc.) due to immune paresis of malignancy
13. Lymphoedema due to lymphatic obstruction by malignancy
14. Generalised hyperhidrosis
15. Necrolytic migratory erythema of glucagonoma
16. Nodular panniculitis (esp. Ca. pancreas)
17. Superficial migratory thrombophebitis (esp. Ca. pancreas)
18. Flush and telangiectasia of malignant carcinoid
19. Bullous pyoderma of leukaemia
20. Bullous eruptions, e.g. pemphigoid (controversial)

FURTHER READING

Sneddon I B 1963 British Medical Journal 2: 405
Staughton R C D 1978 British Journal of Hospital Medicine 20: 38

SCLERODERMA

Scleroderma refers to sclerosis (induration) of the skin and subcutaneous tissue, but some authorities restrict the term to morphoea and systemic sclerosis, and use the term pseudoscleroderma for sclerosis due to other causes

Causes of scleroderma
1. Systemic sclerosis or morphoea
2. Dermatomyositis, LE or rheumatoid disease
3. Cutaneous porphyria
4. Vinyl chloride exposure
5. Chronic gravitational oedema
6. Chronic scurvy (esp. legs)
7. Carcinoid syndrome
8. Mucinous infiltration
   (i)   diffuse myxoedema
   (ii) lichen myxoedematosus
   (iii) scleroedema of Buschke
9. Werner's progeria
10. Graft-versus-host reaction
11. Eosinophilic fasciitis

FURTHER READING

Black Carol 1979 British Journal of Hospital Medicine 22: 28

PORPHYRIA

Simplified synthetic pathway of haem

$$UP\ III \qquad\qquad CP\ III$$
$$\uparrow \qquad\qquad\qquad \uparrow$$

Glycine →ALA→PBG→UPogen III→CPogen III→PP→Haem
succinate

UPogen I ──→ CPogen I

UP I   CP I

Fluorescent

Key: ALA = amino-laevulinic acid
     PBG = porphobilinogen
      UP = uroporphyrin
      CP = corproporphyrin
      PP = protoporphyrin

A specific enzyme defect has now been established in every form of porphyria

HEPATIC PORPHYRIAS

A. Genetic autosomal dominant
1. *Acute intermittent porphyria* (*AIP*)
Classical triad of dark urine, abdominal pain and neuropsychiatric symptoms. May be nausea, constipation, tachycardia, electrolyte disturbances and pigmentation but *no* frank photosensitivity.
Acute attacks precipitated by drugs (barbiturates, sulphonamides, choloroquine, oestrogen and griseofulvin)

Lab.
  (i) Urine darkens on standing and may fluoresce pink under UV radiation
  (ii) Watson-Schwartz Test +ve
    2 ml urine + 2ml Enrlich's aldehyde reagent + 4 ml saturated sodium acetate soln. A purple colour is due to *porphobilinogen* or urobilinogen, but urobilinogen is soluble in chloroform
  (iii) Urinary ALA and PBG are markedly increased, but porphyrins are normal or only slightly increased

2. *Porphyria variegata*
Clinical features of both AIP and PCT

3. *Hereditary coproporphyria*
Rare, resembles AIP

B. Porphyria cutanea tarda (PCT)
Photosensitivity, skin fragility, pigmentation and hirsutism

The genetic enzyme defect (hepatic uroporphyrinogen decarboxylase) is probably expressed only when the liver is damaged, particularly by iron. Most patients are middle-aged alcoholics, but hexachlorobenzene poisoning and hepatic neoplasm can also cause PCT

Lab.
  (i) Urine fluoresces pink, due to increased UP III and CP III
  (ii) Faecal CP III increased
  (iii) Raised Se iron

ERYTHROPOIETIC PORPHYRIAS

1. Congenital erythropoietic porphyria (Gunther's disease)
Very rare defect in haem synthesis characterised by pink teeth, hypertrichosis and severe photosensitivity leading to multilating ulceration. May be haemolytic anaemia and splenomegaly

2. Erythrohepatic proto-porphyria
(Formerly called erythropoietic proto-porphyria)
A familial syndrome with a variety of photosensitivity changes, and burning pain characteristically relieved by cold running water. Also superficial linear scars (pseudorhagades)

Lab.
    (i) Erythrocyte PP is invariably increased
    (ii) Urinary porphyrins normal

Diagnosis of the porphyrias
Remember that:
1. In an acute porphyric attack, the fresh urine may be normal colour and non-fluorescent
2. Urine tests are unreliable for the detection of cutaneous porphyrias, and examination of blood and faeces is necessary

Causes of coproporphyrinuria other than porphyria
1. Alcohol abuse
2. Lead poisoning
3. Liver disease or biliary obstruction
4. Lymphoma, pernicious anaemia, infectious mononucleosis

FURTHER READING

Brodie M J et al 1977 Lancet 2: 699
Goldberg A, McColl K E 1978 Medicine, 3rd series, 11: 551
Kushner J P 1982 New England Journal of Medicine 306: 799

LIPOPROTEINS

Electrophoretic strip

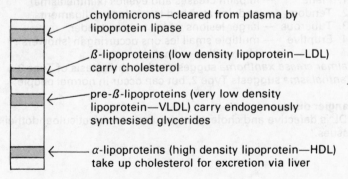

chylomicrons—cleared from plasma by lipoprotein lipase

ß-lipoproteins (low density lipoprotein—LDL) carry cholesterol

pre-ß-lipoproteins (very low density lipoprotein—VLDL) carry endogenously synthesised glycerides

α-lipoproteins (high density lipoprotein—HDL) take up cholesterol for excretion via liver

Hyperlipoproteinaemia (Fredrickson's classification)

Type 1. Familial hyperchylomicronaemia
Presents in childhood as severe hyperlipaemia. Very rare

Type 2. Hyperbeta-lipoproteinaemia of normal density
May be primary (familial hypercholesterolaemia) or secondary to
myxoedema, cholestasis or nephrotic syndrome

Type 3. Hyperbeta-lipoproteinaemia of low density
Usually genetic

Type 4. Hyperprebeta-lipoproteinaemia
A common abnormality secondary to metabolic disease such as
diabetes mellitus, obesity, alcoholism, pancreatitis and nephrotic
syndrome

Type 5. 'Mixed'
Increased chylomicrons and pre-β-lipoproteins
May be genetic or secondary to diabetes or pancreatitis

Conditions associated with severe hyperlipoproteinaemia
1. Ischaemic heart disease
2. Peripheral atheroma
3. Xanthoma
4. Pancreatitis
5. Lipaemia retinalis
6. Hepatosplenomegaly
7. Gout
8. Tendinitis
9. Aortic stenosis

Clinical types of xanthomas
1. Plane   — in palm creases and eyelids (xanthelasma)
2. Tendon   — nodules attached to tendons or ligaments
3. Tuberous — larger lesions which may be tender
4. Eruptive   — multiple small lesions occurring in 'showers',
                        often with a red halo
Palmar crease xanthoma suggests either cholestasis of Type 3
Xanthelasma suggests Type 2, but can occur in normal people

Tangier disease
HDL is defective and cholesterol accumulates in reticuloendothelial
tissues.

FURTHER READING

Chait A Brunzell J D 1981 Medicine International 1: 359
Lewis B 1976 The hyperlipidaemias. Blackwell, Oxford
Thompson G 1978 Medicine, 3rd series, 11: 558

CAUSES OF PHOTOSENSITIVITY

1. *Circulating photosensitisers*
   (i) Albinism and vitiligo
   (ii) Drugs
      Phenothiazines
      Diuretics
      Oral antidiabetics
      Tetracyclines (esp. demethylchlortetracycline)
      Nalidixic acid
      Sulphonamides
      Benoxaprofen
2. *Contact photosensitisers*
   (i) Tar products
   (ii) Furocoumarins (perfumes and plants)
   (iii) Chemicals in soaps and bleaches
3. *Idiopathic dermatoses*
   (i) Photosensitive eczema and actinic reticuloid
   (ii) Polymorphic light eruption
   (iii) Hydroa vacciniforme
   (iv) Solar urticaria
4. *Lack of protection from UVR* (decreased melanin in skin)
   (i) Albinism and vitiligo
   (ii) Phenylketonuria
   (iii) Hypopituitarism
5. *Metabolic defect*
   (i) Pellagra
   (ii) Hartnup disease
6. *Rare congenital diseases*
e.g. Xeroderma pigmentosum, poikiloderma congenitale, etc.

UVR may also precipitate or exacerbate other dermatoses such as LE, herpes simplex and rosacea

FURTHER READING

Magnus I A 1976 Dermatological photosensitivity: Clinical and experimental aspects. Blackwell Scientific, Oxford

PIGMENTATION

CAUSES OF DIFFUSE HYPERPIGMENTATION

1. **Congenital**
   (i) Racial or genetic
   (ii) Fanconi's syndrome (pancytopenia with multiple congenital defects)
2. **Physical agents**
   (i) Radiation, e.g. UVR
   (ii) Chronic rubbing, e.g. 'vagabond's itch'
3. **Post-inflammatory**, e.g. erythroderma
4. **Endocrine**
   (i) Pregnancy, oral contraceptives
   (ii) Hypoadrenalism
   (iii) Acromegaly
   (iv) Hyperthyroidism
   (v) Phaeochromocytoma
   (vi) ACTH therapy or ectopic ACTH from carcinoma
5. **Cachexia of any cause** (esp. malignancy)
6. **Chronic infection**
   Especially malaria, kala-azar, TB, bacterial endocarditis
7. **Nutritional deficiency**
   (i) Malabsorption (esp. sprue)
   (ii) Isolated A, C, B$_{12}$ or folate deficiency
   (iii) Pellagra
8. **Hepatic disease** (esp. biliary cirrhosis, haemochromatosis and hepatolenticular degeneration)
9. **Chronic renal failure**
10. **Collagen-vascular disease**
    (i) Systemic sclerosis
    (ii) Juvenile RA (Still's)
    (iii) Dermatomyositis
    (iv) SLE
11. **Cutaneous porphyria**
12. **Drugs and chemicals**
    (i) Arsenicals
    (ii) Busulphan
    (iii) ACTH
    (iv) Oestrogens
    (v) Chlorpromazine
    (vi) Chloroquine
    (vii) Photodynamic agents, e.g. psoralens

13. **Pigmentation not due to melanin**
    (i) Jaundice—yellow
    (ii) Carotenaemia—yellow
    (iii) Mepacrine—yellow
    (iv) Ochronosis (alkaptanuria)—blue-black
    (v) Argyria (due to silver)—slate-grey
    (vi) Chrysiasis (due to gold)—blue-grey
    (vii) Haemosiderosis (due to iron)—red-brown

FURTHER READING

MacKie Rona 1977 British Journal of Hospital Medicine 17: 48

CAUSES OF HYPOMELANOSIS (MELANIN DEFICIENCY)

A. Circumscribed depigmented patches

Congenital
1. Piebaldism (partial albinism)
2. Waardenburg's syndrome (characteristic facies, with deafness and a white forelock)
3. Tuberose sclerosis (epiloia)
4. Naevus depigmentosus

Acquired
1. Post-inflammatory
    (i) Pityriasis alba
    (ii) Eczema, esp. in Negro
    (iii) Scarring, e.g. burns, varicella
2. Infection
    (i) Pityriasis versicolor
    (ii) Pinta
    (iii) Leprosy
3. Immunological
    (i) Vitiligo
    (ii) Halo naevus (with circulating anti-melanoma antibody)
    (iii) Malignant melanoma
4. Toxins
    (i) Hydroquinones
    (ii) Phenolic germicides

(*contd*)

B. Generalized diffuse hypomelanosis

Congenital
1. Albinism
2. Phenylketonuria
3. Chediak-Higashi syndrome

Acquired
Hypopituitarism

FURTHER READING

Bleehen S S 1974 In: Ledingham J G G (ed) Advanced medicine, symposium 10. Pitman, London, p 317

Conditions associated with vitiligo
1. Organ-specific auto-immune disease
   (i) Thyroiditis
   (ii) Adrenalitis
   (iii) Pernicious anaemia
   (iv) Juvenile-onset diabetes mellitus
2. Alopecia areata
3. Morphea
4. Halo naevus (Sutton's naevus)
5. Malignant melanoma
6. Sunburn and skin cancer

HIRSUTISM

Growth in the female of coarse terminal hair in the male adult sexual pattern.

CAUSES

1. **Idiopathic**
A heterogenous group which includes racial and familial variation. In some cases there is excessive androgen production, usually ovarian, but sometimes adrenal.

2. **Ovarian diseases**
   (i) Polycystic ovaries
       The full Stein-Leventhal syndrome (obesity, amenorrhoea, sterility, polycystic ovaries but no virilization) is relatively rare, but partial forms are much commoner
   (ii) Postmenopausal ovarian stromal hyperplasia
   (iii) Ovarian hilus-cell hyperplasia
   (iv) Ovarian virilizing tumours, e.g. androblastoma
   (v) Gonadal dysgenesis

3. **Adrenal disease**
    (i) ACTH-dependant cortical hyperplasia
        Cushing's
        Ectopic ACTH syndrome
    (ii) Adrenal tumours
    (iii) Late-onset congenital adrenal hyperplasia (C21 or
        11β-hydroxylase defect)

4. **Androgenic drugs**
    Anabolic steroids
    Progestogens

FURTHER READING

Chapman M G 1981 British Journal of Hospital Medicine 26: 270
Vermeulen A 1981 Medicine International 1: 297

HYPERTRICHOSIS

Excessive hair growth in any site

Causes of generalised hypertrichosis
1. Cachexia, especially in children
2. Hereditary diseases
    e.g. erythrohepatic porphyria
        epidermolysis bullosa
        Cornelia de Lange syndrome
        trisomy E
        Hurler's syndrome
3. Head injury, especially in children
4. Dermatomyositis
5. Drugs
    (i) Phenytoin
    (ii) Glucocorticoids
    (iii) Diazoxide, minoxidil
6. Hypertrichosis lanuginosa
    This may be congenital or secondary to internal malignancy

FURTHER READING

Rook A 1972 In: Rook A, Wilkinson D S, Ebling F J G (eds) Textbook of
    dermatology, 2nd edn. Blackwell, Oxford, p 1575

NAILS

Causes of white bands in the nails
1. Fungal infection
2. Chronic hypoalbuminaemia
3. Renal failure
4. Hodgkin's lymphoma
5. Sickle-cell disease
6. Malaria or leprosy
7. Toxins—cytotoxic drugs, arsenic
8. Darier's disease (longitudinal)
9. Congenital leukonychia

Causes of blue or black bands in the nails
1. Subungual haematoma
2. Melanoma
3. Infection by Candida or Pseudomonas
4. Drugs—Chloroquine, cytotoxics
5. Hepatolenticular degeneration (blue lunulae)

FURTHER READING

Samman P D 1972 In: Rook A, Wilkinson D S, Ebling F J G (eds) Textbook of dermatology, 2nd edn. Blackwell, Oxford, p 1642

CLINICAL PATTERNS OF DRUG ERUPTIONS
1. *Exanthemata* (scarlatiniform, morbilliform, papular, etc.)
   Barbiturates, antibiotics, chloral hydrate, etc.
2. *Urticaria*
   Penicillin, salicylates, etc.
3. *Exfoliative dermatitis* (erythroderma)
   Barbiturates, arsenicals, heavy metals, etc.
4. *Fixed eruptions*
   Barbiturates, sulphonamides, phenolphthalein
5. *Bullous eruptions*
   (i) Bromides, iodides, barbiturates, etc.
   (ii) Erythema multiforme (including Stevens-Johnson syndrome) and toxic epidermal necrolysis: Sulphonamides, barbiturates, etc.
   (iii) Pemphigus: Penicillamine
6. *Purpura*
   (i) Drugs causing aplastic anaemia (p. 84)
   (ii) Selective thrombocytopenia: Sedormid, quinine
   (iii) Vascular: carbromal, glucocorticoids, penicillin, etc.
7. *Photo-sensitivity* (toxicity or allergy) (p. 191)

8. *Erythema nodosum*
   Sulphonamides
9. *Acneiform*
   Glucocorticoids, androgens, iodides, bromides, INAH, anticonvulsants, cyanocobalamin
10. *Lichenoid*
    Antimalarials, chlorothiazide, amiphenazole, gold
11. *Pigmentation* (p. 192)
12. *Hypertrichosis* (p. 195) *or hirsutism* (p. 194)
13. *Ichthyosis*
    Nicotinic acid, triparanol
14. *Eczema*
    Systemic administration of a drug after allergic contact dermatitis to the drug has developed
15. *Seborrhoeic dermatitis*
    Methyldopa
16. *SLE-like syndrome*
    Procainamide, hydrallazine, hydantoins, sulphonamides, etc.
17. *Psoriasiform*
    Practolol (also causes eye lesions, otitis media, sclerosing peritonitis, pleurisy and pericarditis)
18. *Livedo reticularis.* Amantadine
19. *Exacerbation of pre-existing skin disease*
    Porphyria—sulphonamides, barbiturates, chloroquine, oestrogens, griseofulvin
    Psoriasis—chloroquine, lithium

PRURITUS

Systemic causes of generalisd pruritus
1. *Hepatic*
   Obstructive jaundice
   Recurrent pruritus of pregnancy
2. *Chronic renal failure* (may be due to secondary hyperparathyroidism)
3. *Blood*
   Malignant lymphoma
   Myeloproliferative disorders (p. 89)
   Fe-deficiency
   Mastocytosis
4. *Carcinoma*, especially lung, stomach, colon, breast
5. *Endocrine*
   Myxoedema or hyperthyroidism
   Carcinoid
6. *Drugs*
   Cocaine, morphine, stilbamidine
   Allergic drug reactions

(contd)

7. *Parasites*: roundworm, trichiniasis, onchocerciasis, etc.
8. *Neurological*
   Tabes or GPI
   Multiple sclerosis
9. *Psychogenic*

Causes of severe pruritus due to skin disease
1. Mites (including scabies), insect bites, pediculosis
2. Eczema
3. Urticaria
4. Lichen planus
5. Dermatitis herpetiformis
6. Lichen simplex chronicus
7. Miliaria rubra (prickly heat)

Causes of palmar erythema
1. Dermatoses, e.g.
   eczema,
   tinea
   psoriasis
   pityriasis rubra pilaris
2. Increased oestrogens
   (i) Pregnancy
   (ii) Cirrhosis, especially alcoholic
3. Arthritis, especially rheumatoid
4. Shoulder-hand syndrome
5. Polycythaemia
6. Beri-beri
7. Mitral insufficiency
8. Diabetes mellitus

INDUSTRIAL SKIN DISEASES
1. **Contact dermatitis**
   (i) Due to irritants
      e.g. cutting oils
         caustics
         organic solvents
         detergents
         fibreglass
         physical factors, etc.
   (ii) Due to allergies
      e.g. chromate in cement, anti-rust paint, leather, etc.
         cobalt in cutting tools, polyester paints, etc.
         nickel in coins, jewellery, cleansing fluids, etc.
         epoxy resins in plastics, electrical components, etc.
         rubber chemicals (vulcanisers, accelerants and
         antioxidants) in tyres, hoses, couplings, etc.

2. **Leukoderma (depigmentation)**
   Due to hydroquinone derivatives, e.g. in adhesives
3. **Industrial acne**
   (i) Folliculitis due to mineral oils
   (ii) Chloracne due to halogenated hydrocarbons
       e.g. dioxin
4. **Skin cancer**
   Due to chronic exposure to tar, mineral oils or chloroprene
5. **Scleroderma (p. 187)**
   Vinyl chloride disease (also causes Raynaud's, pulmonary
   fibrosis, acro-osteolysis and hepatic angio-sarcoma)
6. **Porphyria cutanea tarda**
   Due to dioxin
7. **Fluoride spots**
   Pigmented spots due to atmospheric fluoride from
   aluminium smelting
8. **Lichen planus**
   Due to colour film developers
9. **Chrome ulcers**

FURTHER READING

Rycroft R J G, Calnan C D 1976 British Journal of Hospital Medicine 15: 457

Venereology

PRESENTATION OF GONORRHOEA
1. **Primary genital infection**
   (i) Asymptomatic 'contact'
   (ii) Urethritis
   (iii) Vaginitis or cervicitis
2. **Extension of infection within genital tract**
   Female: endometritis, salpingitis, cystitis, etc.
   Male: prostatitis, cystitis, epididymitis, etc.
3. **Extra-genital dissemination**
   (i) Bacteraemia, may produce rigors or may be asymptomatic
   (ii) Arthritis-dermatitis syndrome:
      Papulo-pustular rash
      Tenosynovitis
      Arthralgia
      Myalgia
      Pyrexia
   (iii) Mono-articular septic joint
   (iv) Endocarditis, myocarditis or pericarditis
   (v) Hepatitis or peri-hepatitis
   (vi) Meningitis
   (vii) Pelvic peritonitis (in female)
4. **Primary extra-genital infection**
   (i) Conjunctivitis or ophthalmitis in neonates
   (ii) Skin infection, stomatitis, pharyngitis, proctitis, etc.
5. **Complications of the above**
   e.g. sterility after salpingitis
        stricture after urethritis

SEROLOGICAL TESTS FOR SYPHILIS

A. **Tests for reagin or antilipoidal Ab**
   Cardiolipin WR
   VDRL slide test (flocculation). May give false negatives
B. **Tests for group-reactive antitrepomenal AB**
   Reiter protein complement fixation. May give false positives

C. **Specific trepomenal tests**
  (i)   Treponemal immobilization test
  (ii) T. pallidum immune adherence
  (iii) Fluorescent trepomenal Ab test (FTA—ABS)
  (iv) T. pallidum haemagglutination TPHA test

Choice of test
  1. **Early syphilis**
    (i) *Primary.* All serology is initially negative, except FTA—ABS
         which may be positive in 80% (useful for male
         homosexuals)
    (ii) *Secondary.* All serology positive
  2. **Late** (2 years post infection)
      Reagin tests may occasionally be negative but specific tests
      with trepomenal Ag tests are positive
In practice the needs of both clinical disease and screening (e.g.
blood donors or antenatal women) can be met by a combination of
tests for reagin (VDRL) and a specific test (TPHA)

FURTHER READING

Oates J K 1979 British Journal of Hospital Medicine 21: 612

Causes of a positive WR
  1. Infections
    (i) Syphilis or yaws
    (ii) Occasionally after vaccinia, infective hepatitis, infectious
         mononucleosis, mycoplasma, malaria, leprosy,
         trypanosomiasis, etc.
  2. Collagen-vascular disease, esp. SLE and Sjøgren's disease
  3. Auto-immune thyroiditis (Hashimoto's)
  4. Auto-immune haemolytic anaemia
  5. Dysproteinaemia
  6. Narcotic addiction
  7. Normal old age
The administration of penicillin to patients with a chronic biological
false positive reaction (BFP) may be dangerous because of their
increased risk of hypersensitivity.

FURTHER READING

Catterall R D 1973 In: Walker G (ed) Advanced medicine, symposium 9.
  Pitman, London, p 97

SECONDARY SYPHILIS

Clinical features
1. Tiredness, fever, myalgia, sore throat and headache (often worst at night)
2. Slight lymphadenopathy
3. A polymorphous maculo-papular rash. Commonly involves palms and soles and is rarely irritable or vesicular.
4. Condyloma lata of anus and genitalia
5. Mucous patches of mouth, pharynx or larynx
6. Patchy alopecia ('glades in the wood')
7. Less commonly hepatitis, iritis, arthritis, periostitis or neuritis may occur

N.B. Must be considered in any atypical dermatosis

FURTHER READING

Thin R N 1978 Medicine, 3rd series, 6: 268.

Immunology

Allergy means the specifically altered state of reactivity of a host following exposure to an allergen. The term applies to either hypersensitivity or immunity

Classification of harmful allergic reactions

Type I. Anaphylactic

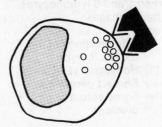

▲ Antigen (Ag)
< Antibody (Ab)

Reaginic Ab (IgE) bound to tissue cells (e.g. mast cells) causes release of vasoactive substances on contact with Ag
Examples
    (i) Anaphylaxis
    (ii) Hay-fever, urticaria, asthma

Type II. Cytotoxic

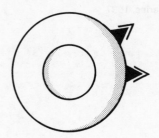

Ab (usually IgG or IgM) reacts with Ag bound to cell surface. This often involves complement fixation and cell damage
Examples
    (i) Blood transfusion reactions
    (ii) Haemolytic disease of the newborn
    (iii) Auto-allergic harmolytic anaemia
    (iv) Post-streptococcal glomerulonephritis

Type III. Circulating immune complex (Arthus)

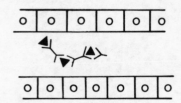

Free Ag and Ab combine and in certain conditions the complexes precipitate, with complement fixation and damage to small bloodvessels
Example
Serum sickness

Type IV: Cell-mediated (Delayed hypersensitivity)

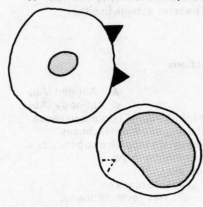

Sensitised lymphocytes react with Ag deposited at a local site and release lymphokines such as mitogenic factor and macrophage migration inhibition factor. Probably involves cooperation between T and B lymphocytes and macrophages
Examples
    (i) Skin reactions of the tuberculin type
   (ii) Homograft rejection
  (iii) Contact dermatitis
  (iv) Some auto-allergic diseases

FURTHER READING

Holborow J, Lessof M 1978 Medicine, 3rd, series, 1: 37

T AND B LYMPHOCYTES

Distinctions between T and B lymphocytes

	T cells	B cells
Ig on cell surface	Absent or not easily demonstrated	Easily demonstrated
Fc receptors	Absent	Present
Complement receptors	Absent	Present
Sheep RBC binding to form rosettes	Yes	No
Response to mitogens—		
Phytohaemaglutinin	Yes	No
Conconavilin-A	Yes	No

FURTHER READING

McConnell I 1976 In: Peters D K (ed) Advanced medicine, symposium 12. Pitman, London, p 1

B LYMPHOCYTE DEFICIENCIES

A. Primary

Hypogammaglobulinaemia
1. Congenital sex-linked (Bruton's)
2. Non-sex-linked agammaglobulinaemia
3. Hypogammaglobulinaemia of late onset
4. Combined immunodeficiency syndromes
    (i) Alymphocytic (Swiss-type)
    (ii) Thymic dysplasia
    (iii) Achondroplastic

Dysgammaglobulinaemia (normal γ-globulin on electrophoresis)
Types I to VII, e.g. selective deficit of IgA (Type IV) occurs in ataxia telangiectasia, and selective deficit of IgM (Type V) in Wiskott-Aldrich syndrome

B. Secondary
1. *Defective synthesis*
    (i) Prematurity or delayed maturity
    (ii) Lymphoma, myelomatosis or Waldenström's macroglobulinaemia
    (iii) Marrow disorders, e.g. myelosclerosis, metastases, hypoplasia
    (iv) Irradiation and cytotoxic drugs

(contd)

2. *Protein deficiency*
    (i) Nephrotic syndrome
    (ii) Protein-losing enteropathy
    (iii) Severe malnutrition or malabsorption
    (iv) Exfoliative dermatitis
    (v) Myotonic dystrophy

Causes of hypergammaglobulinaemia
1. *Diffuse 'broad band' type* (polyclonal gammopathy)
    (i) Chronic infection
    (ii) Hepatic disease
    (iii) 'Collagen vascular' disease, also ulcerative colitis, Crohn's, Hashimoto's thyroiditis, etc.
2. *Narrow 'M band' type* (monoclonal gammopathy)
    (i) Multiple myeloma
    (ii) Waldenström's macroglobulinaemia
    (iii) 'Benign' paraproteinaemia, especially in old people
    (iv) Heavy chain disease (May be γ μ or α)
    (v) Bence-Jones proteinuria in absence of myelomatosis
    (vi) Leukaemia, lymphoma or carcinoma
    (vii) Primary cold agglutinins
    (viii) Amyloidosis
    (ix) Lichen myxoedematosus

T LYMPHOCYTE DEFICIENCIES

A. Primary
1. Thymic and parathyroid aplasia (Di George's)
2. Lymphopenia with normal immunoglobulins (Nezelof's)
3. Episodic lymphopenia with lymphocytotoxin
4. Qualitative lymphocyte defects (e.g. chronic mucocutaneous Candidosis)

B. Secondary
1. Malignancy, esp. T cell lymphoma
2. Various (? immunological) diseases, e.g. eczema, multiple sclerosis
3. Kwashiorkor
4. Secondary to B cell deficiency

FURTHER READING

Hayward, A. (1975) In: Taylor G (ed) Immunology in medical practice. Saunders, London, p 33
Hobbs J R 1974 In: Hardisty R M, Weatherall D J (eds) Blood and its disorders, Blackwell, Oxford, p 1319

CAUSES OF PHAGOCYTE DYSFUNCTION

1. **Defective chemotaxis**
    (i) Diabetes mellitus
    (ii) Steroid therapy
    (iii) Malnutrition
    (iv) Malignancy, esp. Hodgkin's disease
    (v) Renal failure
    (vi) Severe burns
    (viii) SLE and rheumatoid disease
    (ix) Granulomata (Sarcoid, Crohn's)
    (x) Some antibiotics, esp. tetracycline
    (xi) Lazy leucocyte syndrome
2. **Defective opsonisation**
    (i) Complement deficiency, e.g. C3 or C5
    (ii) IgM deficiency (e.g. in neonates)
    (iii) Sickle-cell anaemia
    (vi) Absence of spleen
    (v) SLE
3. **Defective intracellular bacterial killing**
    (i) Chronic granulomatous disease of childhood
        Lymphadenopathy, hepatomegaly, pneumonia, dermatitis, abscesses, osteomyelitis. Due to defective hydrogen peroxide production
    (ii) Job's syndrome
        Recurrent cold staphylococcal abscesses
    (iii) Chediak-Higashi syndrome
        Partial oculo-cutaneous albinism. Giant lysosomes in granulocytes. Recurrent bacterial infections, sometimes with a lymphomatoid reaction
    (iv) Myeloperoxidase deficiency
    (v) Severe glucose-6-P dehydrogenase deficiency
    (vi) Drugs
        Glucocorticoids colchicine, etc.

FURTHER READING

Johnston R B 1982 New England Journal of Medicine 307: 434
Segal A W 1980 Hospital Update 6: 1043
Smith C 1978 Medicine, 3rd series, 4: 187

COMPLEMENT

SOME INHERITED COMPLEMENT DEFECTS ASSOCIATED WITH CLINICAL EFFECTS

Deficiency	Association
C1 inhibitor	Hereditary angio-oedema, due to unrestrained complement activation
C1r	
C1s	SLE-like syndrome
C2	'Immune-complex' disease
	Henoch-Schönlein purpura, glomerulonephritis, SLE, etc.
C3	Recurrent infections
Terminal components,	
C5-C9	Recurrent infections (esp. Neisseria)

FURTHER READING

Lachmann P J In: Peters D K (ed) Advanced medicine, vol 12. Pitman, London, p 43
Haeney M (1982) Hospital Update 8: 289

Skin testing for immunological reactions
Type I (*Prick test*) an urticarial wheal, developing within 20 minutes and resolving within 2 hours
Type III (*ID injection*) an ill-defined red swelling, sometimes purpuric, developing over several hours, maximal at 5–7 hours and resolving in 24–36 hours
Type IV (*ID injection or Patch test*) an indurated red area, sometimes with vesiculation, developing within 24–48 hours and resolving over several days

FURTHER READING

Pepys J 1975 British Journal of Hospital Medicine 14: 412

Genetics

GLOSSARY OF TERMS

Alleles. Alternative forms of a gene occupying the same locus on homologous chromosomes. A child should receive one of each pair of alleles from each parent

Aneuploid. A chromosome number which is not an exact multiple of the haploid number

Autosome. Any chromosome other than the sex chromosomes. Man has 22 pairs of autosomes

Barr body. The sex chromatin seen in somatic cells of the female

Carrier. An individual who is hererozygous for a normal gene and an abnormal gene which is not expressed phenotypically

Chimera. An individual composed of cells from different zygotes. In 'blood-group' chimerism dyzygotic twins exchange haemopoietic stem cells in utero and continue to form blood cells of both types. In 'whole-body' chimerism two separate zygotes are fused into one individual

Chromatid. A chromosome consists of two parallel strands (chromatids) held together by the centromere

Clone. A cell line derived by mitosis from a single ancestral diploid cell

Concordant. A term used to describe a pair of twins in which both members exhibit a certain trait

Crossover. Exchange of genetic material between members of a chromosome pair

Deletion. A chromosomal aberration in which part of a chromosome is lost

Diploid. The number of chromosomes in somatic cells (which is double that of the gametes). In man this is 46

Discordant. A term used to describe a pair of twins in which one shows a certain trait and the other does not

Dizygotic. Twins produced by two ova, separately fertilised

Duplication. a chromosomal aberration in which part of a chromosome is duplicated

F1. The first generation progeny of a mating

Gametes. Reproductive cells which unite in pairs to form a zygote

Gene. A segment of DNA coded for the synthesis of a single polypeptide

Genome. (Genotype) The full set of genes

Haploid. The chromosome number of a normal gamete. In man this is 23

Hemizygous. A term applied to genes on the X chromosome in a male

Heterogeneity. A phenotype is genetically heterogeneous if it can be produced by different genetic mechanisms

Heterozygote. An individual with 2 different alleles at a given locus on a pair of homologous chromosomes

Holandric. The inheritance pattern of genes on a Y chromosome (i.e. transmitted to all sons but no daughters)

Homologous chromosomes. A 'matched pair' of chromosomes, one from each parent, having the same gene loci in the same order

Homozygote. An individual with 2 identical alleles at a given locus on a pair of homologous chromosomes

Inversion. A chromosomal aberration in which a segment of chromosome is inverted end-to-end

Isoalleles. 'Normal' alleles which can be distinguished from each other only by their differing phenotypic expression when in combination with a dominant mutant allele

Isochromosome. An abnormal chromosome with 2 arms of equal length, bearing the same loci in reverse sequence, formed by transverse (instead of longitudinal) division of the centromere

Karyotype. The chromosome set

Locus. The position of a gene on a chromosome

Mosaic. An individual or tissue with at least 2 cell lines differing in genotype

Multiple alleles. More than 2 alleles may occur at a given locus in a population even though each normal individual can have only 2 alleles at that locus

Penetrance. The frequency of expression of a genotype. A non-penetrant trait is not expressed in the phenotype

Phenotype. The individual produced by the interaction between the genotype and the environment

Pleiotropy. The production of multiple effects by a single gene

Polygenic. Determined by many genes at different loci, with small additive effects

Proband. (Propositus, index case.) The family member who first presents with a given trait

Recombination. The formation of new combinations of linked genes by crossing over between their loci

RNA. Ribonucleic acid, has 3 forms:

   (i)   messenger RNA is the template for polypeptide synthesis
   (ii) transfer RNA brings activated amino-acids into position along this template
   (iii) ribosomal RNA is a component of ribosomes which functions as a non-specific site of polypeptide synthesis

Segregation.. The separation of allelic genes at meiosis

Sex chromatin. (Barr body) A chromatin mass in the nucleus which represents an inactive X chromosome. It is absent in the male

Sex-limited. A trait expressed only in one sex though the gene determining it is not X-linked

Sex-linked. A trait expressed by a gene on the X chromosome

Synteny. The presence of 2 or more gene loci on the same chromosome

Triplet. 3 successive bases in DNA or RNA which code for a specific amino-acid

Triploid. A cell or individual with 3 times the normal haploid chromosome number

Trisomy. The presence of 3 of a given chromosome instead of the usual pair, as in trisomy 21 (Down's)

Zygote. The fertilised ovum

FURTHER READING

Emery A E H 1975 Elements of medical genetics, 4th edn. Churchill Livingstone, Edinburgh
Thompson, J, Thompson M 1973 Genetics in medicine. Saunders, Philadelphia, p 357

HISTOCOMPATIBILITY (HL-A) ANTIGENS

Histocompatibility antigens are present on all tissues of the body.
There are two series of antigens determined serologically at each of
2 loci, and a further series of antigens determined only in the mixed
lymphocyte reaction. Some diseases occur more frequently in
association with certain HL-A antigens, possibly due to related
immune response (IR) genes.

The strongest association is between ankylosing spondylitis and
B27

The following 'immunological' diseases are associated with B8:
1. Active chronic hepatitis
2. SLE
3. Sjøgren's disease
4. Juvenile dermatomyositis
5. Dermatitis herpetiformis
6. Coeliac disease
7. Graves' disease
8. Myasthenia gravis
9. Juvenile, insulin-dependent, diabetes mellitus
10. Addison's hypoadrenalism

FURTHER READING

Dick Heather 1981 In: Dawson A M, Compston N, Besser G M (eds) Recent
    advances in medicine—18. Churchill Livingstone, Edinburgh, p 1
Sasazuki T et al 1977 Annual Review of Medicine 28: 425
Woodrow J C 1981 Hospital Update 7: 689

Pyrexia and hypothermia

Causes of PUO
1. Infection
   - (i) Exclude:
     tonsillitis, pneumonia, pyelonephritis, cholangitis, enteric fever, septicaemia, pus under tension, endocarditis, pericarditis, etc.
   - (ii) Consider possibility of:
     TB, brucellosis, parasites (worms, malaria, etc.) and viral infections
2. Collagen-vascular disease
3. Malignancy (e.g. hypernephroma, lymphoma, hepatoma or atrial myxoma)
4. 'Silent' myocardial or pulmonary infarction
5. Drug hypersensitivity prior to onset of rash
6. Rarities: Familial Mediterranean fever, Whipple's disease, Fabry's, Weber-Christian, etc.
7. Psychogenic and hysteria
8. Munchausen's syndrome

FURTHER READING

Daggett P 1976 British Journal of Hospital Medicine 16: 357
Munro J 1978 Medicine, 3rd series, 7: 327
Wood M J 1981 Medicine International 1: 24

HYPOTHERMIA

Causes of hypothermia
1. *Decreased heat production*
   - (i) Hypothyroidism or hypopituitarism
   - (ii) Hypoglycaemia or severe malnutrition
   - (iii) Inactivity—crippling disease, Parkinsonism, depression, etc.

(contd)

2. *Increased heat loss*
   (i) Exposure in a cold environment
   (ii) Erythroderma
   (iii) Alcoholic intoxication
   (iv) Paget's disease
3. *Failure of thermoregulation*
   (a) *Central*
   (i) 'Stroke' (especially intra-cranial bleed in infants)
   (ii) Drugs, e.g. barbiturates, phenothiazines
   (iii) Uraemia or diabetic ketoacidosis
   (iv) Moribundity
   (v) Miscellaneous neurological diseases, e.g. Wernicke's encephalopathy, diencephalic epilepsy, craniopharyngioma
   (b) *Peripheral* (autonomic dysfunction)
      Any severe illness

Complications of hypothermia

1. *Pulmonary*
   Bronchopneumonia, pulmonary oedema or hypotension may be induced by fast rewarming
2. *Cardiac*
   Ventricular fibrillation or bradyarrhythmias
3. *Metabolic*
   Hypoxia, hypercapnia, acidosis, hypoglycaemia or fluid shifts
4. *Gastro-intestinal*
   Haemorrhagic erosions, gastric or colonic dilatation, ileus, pancreatitis
5. *Others*
   Disseminated intravascular coagulation
   Microinfarcts in many tissues

FURTHER READING

Emslie-Smith D 1981 British Journal of Hospital Medicine 26: 442
Johnson R H, Spalding J M K 1976 British Journal of Hospital Medicine 15: 266

Microbiology

Gram staining of some important pathogens

Gram +ve
Actinomyces
Anthrax
Clostridia
Coryn. diphtheriae
Pneumococcus
Staphylococcus
Streptococcus
TB

Gram −ve
Brucella
Cholera
E. coli-Salmonella-Shigella
Haemophilus influenzae
Haemophilus pertussis
Klebsiella
Neisseria (gonococcus, meningococcus)
Pasteurella
Pseudomonas
Proteus
Rickettsiae

Bactericidal drugs
Penicillins, cephalosporins
Streptomycin, neomycin
Kanamycin
Co-trimoxazole
Polymyxin, colistin
Isoniazid
Bacitracin
Metronidazole
Aminoglycosides (tobramycin) and gentamycin)

Bacteriostatic drugs
Sulphonamides
Tetracyclines
Chloramphenicol
Erythromycin
Novobiocin
PAS
Lincomycin, clindamycin

Organisms virtually always sensitive to penicillin
Strep. pyogenes (Gp.A)
Strep. pneumoniae (pneumococcus)
Neisseria meningitidis
Treponema pallidum

CLASSIFICATION OF SOME COMMON VIRUSES

RNA containing viruses

1. *Picornaviruses*
   (i) Enteroviruses
       Polio
       Echo
       Coxsackie
   (ii) Rhinoviruses
        Coryza etc.
2. *Myxoviruses and paramyxoviruses*
       Influenza
       Mumps
       Measles
       Respiratory syncytial

3. *Reoviruses*
       Upper respiratory
       tract infections
4. *Arborviruses*
       Endemic encephalitis
       Yellow fever
       Dengue
       Sandfly fever
5. *Rhabdoviruses*
       Rabies

SLOW VIRUS INFECTIONS

1. Subacute sclerosing parencephalitis (usually measles).
2. Progressive multifocal leukoencephalopathy (usually in lymphoma or sarcoidosis).
3. Kuru (probably confined to New Guinea).
4. Creutzfeldt-Jakob disease

FURTHER READING

Matthews W B 1981 Journal of the Royal College of Physicians 15: 109

Incubation periods of some tropical infections

Less than 10 days	Dengue
	Yellow fever
	Tick typhus
	Plague
	Paratyphoid
10 to 21 days	Malaria (prolonged by drugs)
	Lassa fever
	Scrub typhus
	African trypanosomiasis
	Typhoid
More than 21 days	Filariasis
	Leprosy
	Leishmaniasis (cutaneous and visceral)

FURTHER READING

Ree G H 1977 British Journal of Hospital Medicine 17: 38

DNA containing viruses

1. *Poxviruses*
   Variola
   Vaccinia
   Molluscum contagiosum
   Orf
2. *Adenoviruses*
   Upper respiratory tract infections
   Conjunctivitis, etc.
3. *Herpesviruses*
   Herpesvirus hominis (H. simplex)
   Varicella-zoster
   Epstein Barr virus
   Cytomegalic inclusion disease
4. *Papillomaviruses*
   Verruca vulgaris

Clinical chemistry

NORMAL ADULT RANGE FOR LABORATORY ASSAYS

The International System of Units (SI units) has now been widely introduced in British laboratories in place of the traditional Imperial Units, which were empirical. SI units are preferred by the Royal Colleges for examination questions. Submultiples of SI units use the following prefixes:

Factor	Name	Symbol
10^{-1}	deci	d
10^{-2}	centi	c
10^{-3}	milli	m
10^{-6}	micro	μ
10^{-9}	nano	n
10^{-12}	pico	p
10^{-15}	femto	f

Even with SI units, values may vary in different laboratories.

FURTHER READING

Paterson N, Fraser S C 1975 British Journal of Hospital Medicine 13: 757

Blood
Acid phosphatase, 1–3.5 KA units/100 ml
    (Tartrate labile, up to 0.8 KA units/100 ml)
Alanine amino-transferase, up to 45 Reitman-Frankel units/ml
Alkaline phosphatase, 25–85 IU/100 ml (3–13 KA units/100 ml)
Ammonium, 23–47 μmol/l (40–80 μg/100 ml)
Amylase, up to 200 Somogyi units
Ascorbic acid, 34–114 μmol/l (0.6–2.0 mg/100 ml)
Aspartate amino-transferase, up to 50 Reitman-Frankel units/ml
B_{12}, 100–1000 ng/l (or $\mu\mu$g/ml)
Bilirubin (total), up to 17 μmol/l (up to 1 mg/100 ml)
Calcium, 2.2–2.7 mmol/l (9.0–10.8 mg/100 ml)

Ionized calcium, 1.1–2.4 mmol/l (4.5–5.6 mg/100 ml)
Cholesterol, 3.6–6.7 mmol/l (140–260 mg/100 ml)
Cholinesterase, 2–4 units
Copper, 12–25 μmol/l (75–160 μg/100 ml)
Copper oxidase, 0.20–0.55 units
Cortisol, (11-hydroxycorticosteroids)
    9 am, 190–690 nmol/l (7–25 μg/100 ml)
    12 midnight, 80–190 nmol/l (3–7 μg/100 ml)
Creatinine, 53–106 μmol/l (0.6–1.2 mg/100 ml)
Electrolytes
    Na, 136–149 mmol/l (or mEq/l)
    K, 3.8–5.2 mmol/l (or mEq/l)
    Cl, 100–107 mmol/l (or mEq/l)
    Bicarb, 24–30 mmol/l (or mEq/l)
Fibrinogen, 2–4 g/l (200–400 mg/100 ml)
Folate, 6–21 μg/l (or mμg/ml)
Glucose (fasting venous sample, glucose oxidase assay),
    3.0–5.3 mmol/l (55–95 mg/100 ml)
Haptoglobin, 0.7–1.3 g/l (72–125 mg/100 ml)
HGH, 1–5 μIU/ml during G.T.T.
Immunoglobulins
    IgG, 80–160 mg/l
    IgA, 14–42 mg/l
    IgM, 5–19 mg/l
    IgD, 0.03–4 mg/l
Iron
    Males, 14–32 μmol/l (80–180 μg/100 ml)
    Females, 11–29 μmol/l (60–160 μg/100 ml)
Lactic dehydrogenase, 55–200 IU/l (110–400
    spectrophotometric units/ml)
5-Nucleotidase, 1.6–17.0 IU/l
Phosphate, 0.8–1.4 mmol/l (2.5–4.5 mg/100 ml)
Protein (total), 60–80 g/l (6–8 g/100 ml)
    Albumin, 33–46 g/l (3.3–4.6 g/100 ml)
    α1 globulin, 1–4 g/l (0.1–0.4 g/l100 ml)
    α2 globulin, 5–10 g/l (0.5–1.0 g/100 ml)
    β globulin, 6–11 g/l (0.6–1.1 g/100 ml)
    γ globulin; 6–12 g/l (0.6–1.2 g/l100 ml)
Protein-bound iodine, 236–550 nmol/l (3.0–7.0 μg/100 ml)
Red cell folate, 160–640 μg/l (or mμg/ml)
Thymol turbidity, 0–4 units
Thyroxine 70–160 nmol/l
TIBC, 45–72 μmol/l (250–400 μg/100 ml)
Triglycerides (fasting) 0.3–1.7 mmol/l
Urea, 2.5–6.6 mmol/l (15–40 mg/100 ml)
Uric acid, up to 0.4 mmol/l (up to 6 mg/100 ml)

Blood gases (arterial)
Oxygen 12–15 k Pa (90–100 mmHg)
Carbon dioxide 4.5–6.1 k Pa (34–46 mmHg)

Urine (assuming a normal diet)
Specific gravity 1.008–1.030
pH 4.8–7.5
Ascorbic acid, 114–170 μmol/24 h (20–30 mg/24 hr)
Calcium, 2.5–7.5 mmol/24 (100–300 mg/24 hr)
Chloride, 100–180 mmol/24 h (or mEq/24 hr)
Creatinine, 9–17 mmol/24 h (1–2 g/24 hr)
5HIAA, 16–73 μmol/24 h (3–14 mg/24 hr)
Phosphate, 16–48 mmol/24 h (0.5–1.5 g/24 hr)
Potassium, 25–100 mmol/24 h (or mEq/24 hr)
Sodium, 100–200 mmol/24 h (or mEq/24 hr)
VMA, 10–40 μmol/24 h (2–8 mg/24 hr)
17-Hydroxycorticoids (Porter-Silber),
    Male 3–10 mg/24 hr
    Female 2–6 mg/24 hr
17-Ketosteroids,
    Male 9–22 mg/24 hr
    Female 6–15 mg/24 hr
Urea 250–500 mmol/l (10–40 g/24 hr)

CSF
Chloride, 120–128 mmol/l (or mEq/l)
Glucose, 2.5–3.9 mmol/l (45–70 mg/100 ml)
Protein, up to 0.4 g/l (up to 40 mg/100 ml)
Lymphocytes, up to 4/cu mm

FURTHER READING

Keen H, Liddell J 1978 Medicine, 3rd series, 11: 556

SPECIAL TESTS

Glucose tolerance test
Normal limits, using 50 g oral load with capillary samples and reduction method of assay
1. Fasting true blood glucose does not exceed 6.7 mmol/l (120) mg/100 ml)
2. Blood glucose does not rise above 8.9 mmol/l (160 mg/100 ml)
3. Blood glucose returns below 6.7 mmol/l (120 mg/100 ml within 2 hr)

'Maximal' gastric secretion test
Using pentagastrin 6 μg/kg IM

Basal sample (*60 min*)	*Post-pentagastrin samples* (*60 min*)
Females: 1–2 mEq/hr	10–20 mEq/hr
Males: 2–3 mEq/hr	15–25 mEq/hr

Creatinine clearance should exceed 100 ml/min

Ammonium chloride test for urinary acidification
(using 0.1 g/kg body wt of NH_4Cl)
Urine pH should fall below 5.3 and urinary titratable acidity should exceed 25 μEq/min

Phosphate excretion index (PEI)
The ratio $\dfrac{\text{phosphate clearance}}{\text{creatinine clearance}}$ is dependent upon the plasma PO_4 level.

The PEI indicates the extent to which this ratio departs from the predicted normal for a given plasma PO_4 level.

i.e. PEI = Observed $\dfrac{CP}{CCr}$ – 'Normal' $\dfrac{CP}{CCr}$

where the normal $\dfrac{CP}{CCr}$ = 0.055 plasma PO_4 – 0.07.

On a normal diet, PEI should be 0 ± 0.09

BSP excretion test (using 5 mg/kg)
Not more than 5 per cent BSP should remain in the blood at 45 minutes

Xylose absorption test (using 25 g xylose)
The 5 hour urinary excretion of xylose should exceed 6 g

Fat absorption test on normal diet
Total faecal fat over 5 days should not exceed 5 g/day

Dexamethasone suppression test
1. Dexamethasone 0.5 mg 6 hourly for 2 days
   Normally urinary 17-Hydroxycorticoids suppress to less than 2.5 mg/24 hr
   In adrenocortical hyperplasia there is less suppression
2. Dexamethasone 2.0 mg 6 hourly for 2 days
   With bilateral hyperplasia there is suppression to less than 50% of the base-line assay
   With adenoma or carcinoma there is less suppression

Note that exceptions may occur

Synacthen test

Plasma cortisol (11-OHCS) is measured before and 30 min after 250 μg Synacthen IM

The initial cortisol conc should exceed 138 nmol/l (5 μg/100 ml)
At 30 min the cortisol conc should exceed 495 nmol/l (18 μg/100 ml) and the increment (irrespective of the initial level) should exceed 193 nmol/l (7 μg/100 ml)

Insulin tolerance tests (Dangerous in hypopituitarism)

Standard. After an overnight fast, soluble insulin is given IV in a dose of 0.1 U/kg and blood glucose, cortisol and GH are measured every 30 min for 2 hr. GH conc should exceed 10 μIU/ml in at least one post-insulin specimen.

Augmented ITT (for acromegaly) uses 0.3 U/kg and should not be performed if hypopituitarism is suspected

Bibliography

It is unlikely that even the most assiduous of candidates will find time to study all of the following books. Special attention should be paid to the subjects in which the least clinical experience has been gained. It is more important to cover the whole of medicine superficially than to know some subjects in great detail with areas of complete ignorance in other subjects. A thorough knowledge of a small textbook will be more useful than a patchy knowledge of a large one.

It is essential to read a book on the elicitation and interpretation of physical signs, e.g. *Hutchison's Clinical Methods* by Bomford et al or *Clinical Examination* by Macleod. The British National Formulary is also strongly recommended for study.

The following Colour Atlases published by Wolfe Medical and Scientific Publications, London provide a valuable form of vicarious clinical experience:

Bone Disease	(V. Parsons)
Cardiology	(N. Conway)
Clinical Neurology	(M. Parsons)
Dermatology	(G. M. Levene and C. D. Calnan)
Diabetes	(A. Bloom and J. Ireland)
Endocrinology	(R. Hall, D. Evered and R. Greene)
Hand Conditions	(W. B. Connolly)
Infectious Diseases	(R.T.D. Edmond)
Liver Disease	(S. Sherlock and J. Summerfield)
Nutritional Disorders	(D. S. MacLaren)
Ophthalmological Diagnosis	(M. A. Bedford)
Oral Medicine	(W. R. Tyldesley)
Respiratory Diseases	(D. G. James and P. R. Studdy)
Rheumatology	(A. C. Boyle)
Tropical Medicine and Parasitology	(W. Peters and H. M. Gilles)
Venereology	(A. Wisdom)

Asterisks denote larger texts and reference books

Cardiology
Schire V 1977 Clinical cardiology, 3rd edn. Granada, London
*Braunwald E 1980 Heart disease—A textbook of cardiovascular medicine. Saunders, London

Electrocardiography
Schamroth L 1971 An introduction to electrocardiography, 4th edn. Blackwell, Oxford
*Goldman M J 1976 Principles of clinical electrocardiography, 9th edn. Lange, Los Altos

Chest disease
Flenley D C 1981 Respiratory medicine. Bailliere Tindall, London
*Crofton J, Douglas A 1981 Respiratory diseases, 3rd edn. Blackwell, Oxford

Gastro-enterology
Naish J M, Read A E 1974 Basic gastroenterology, 2nd edn. Wright, Bristol
*Sleisenger M H, Fordtran J S 1978 Gastro-intestinal disease, 2nd edn. Saunders, Philadelphia
*Sherlock Sheila 1981 Diseases of the liver and biliary system, 6th edn. Blackwell, Oxford

Haematology
Thompson R B 1975 A short textbook of haematology, 4th edn. Pitman, London
*Pennington D, Bush B, Castaldi P 1978 Clinical haematology in medical practice, 4th edn. Blackwell Scientific, Oxford
Hoffbrand A V, Lewis S M 1981 Postgraduate haematology, 2nd edn. Heinemann, London

Neurology
Walton J N 1975 Essentials of neurology, 4th edn. Pitman, London
*Walton J N 1977 Brain's diseases of the nervous system, 8th edn. Oxford University Press, Oxford
*Merrit H H 1979 A textbook of neurology, 6th edn. Lea & Febiger, Philadelphia
*Walton J 1981 Disorders of voluntary muscles, 4th edn. Churchill Livingstone, Edinburgh

Endocrine and bone disease
Hall R, Anderson J, Smart G A, Besser M 1974 Fundamentals of clinical endocrinology, 2nd edn. Pitman, London
*Toft A D, Campbell W, Seth J 1981 Diagnosis and management of endocrine diseases. Blackwell Scientific, Oxford

*Nordin B E C 1973 Metabolic bone and stone disease. Churchill Livingstone, Edinburgh

Oakley W G, Pyke D A, Taylor K W 1979 Diabetes and its management, 3rd edn. Blackwell Scientific, Oxford

Renal disease

Gabriel R 1978 Postgraduate nephrology, 2nd edn. Butterworth, London

Davison A M 1981 A synopsis of renal diseases. Wright, Bristol

*Strauss M B, Welt L H 1972 Diseases of the kidney, 2nd edn. Churchill Livingstone, Edinburgh

*Black Sir Douglas, Jones A F 1979 Renal disease, 4th edn. Blackwell, Oxford

Rheumatology

Hughes G R V 1979 Connective tissue diseases, 2nd edn. Blackwell, Oxford

Mason M, Currey H L F 1976 An introduction to clinical rheumatology. Pitman Medical, London

*Kelley W N, Harris E D Jr et al 1980 Textbook of rheumatology. Saunders, London

Immunology

Roitt I 1980 Essential immunology, 4th edn. Blackwell, Oxford

Dermatology

Burton J L 1979 Essentials of dermatology. Churchill Livingstone, Edinburgh

*Braverman I M 1981 Skin signs of systemic disease. Saunders, London

*Rook A, Wilkinson D S, Ebling F J G 1979 Textbook of dermatology, 3rd edn. Blackwell, Oxford

Venereology

Noble R C 1979 Sexually transmitted disease. Kimpton, London

Clinical chemistry

Zilva J F, Pannall P R 1979 Clinical chemistry in diagnosis and treatment, 3rd edn. Lloyd-Luke, London

Medical emergencies

Matthew H, Lawson A A H 1979 Treatment of common acute poisonings, 4th edn. Churchill Livingstone, Edinburgh

Baderman H 1978 Management of medical emergencies. Pitman, London

Infectious disease

Ramsay A M, Esmond R T D 1978 Infectious diseases, 2nd edn. Heinemann, London

Radiology
Bretland P M 1978 Essentials of radiology. Butterworth, London
Greenfield G B 1975 Radiology of bone disease, 2nd edn. Blackwell, Oxford

Occupational medicine
Hunter D 1975 The diseases of occupations, 5th edn. English Universities Press, London

General
Bomford R R, Mason S, Swash M 1975 Hutchison's clinical methods, 16th edn. Bailliere Tindall, London
Burton J L 1980 Aids to undergraduate medicine, 3rd edn. Churchill Livingstone, Edinburgh
Davies I J T 1977 Postgraduate medicine, 3rd edn. Lloyd-Luke, London
Gabriel R, Gabriel Cynthia 1978 Medical data interpretation for MRCP. Butterworth, London
Macleod J 1979 Clinical examination, 5th edn. Churchill Livingstone, Edinburgh
Spalton D J, Sever P S, Ward P D 1976 100 case histories for the MRCP. Churchill Livingstone, Edinburgh
*Isselbacher K J et al 1980 Harrison's principles of internal medicine. McGraw Hill, New York

JOURNALS

Excellent review articles suitable for M.R.C.P. candidates appear regularly in Medicine, Hospital Update and the British Journal of Hospital Medicine. Relevant leading articles in the British Medical Journal, The Lancet and the New England Journal of Medicine should also be read. These latter journals also contain many important original papers, and though one cannot read every paper in detail it is worth scanning each issue to pick out important advances relating to internal medicine. Every reader must develop a method which suits him best, but I find that the quickest way to imprint the 'message' of a paper on my memory is to read the Summary, then the Introduction (which puts the work in perspective and explains why it was done) and then re-read the Summary. Examination candidates are unlikely to have time to read the Methods and Discussion of original papers except in subjects in which they have a special interest.

It is worth remembering that many M.R.C.P. examiners regularly read the Quarterly Journal of Medicine.

Index